THE POLITICS OF REPRODUCTION IN OTTOMAN SOCIETY, 1838–1900

The Body, Gender and Culture

Series Editor: *Lynn Botelho*

Titles in this Series

1 Courtly Indian Women in Late Imperial India
Angma Dey Jhala

2 Paracelsus's Theory of Embodiment: Conception and Gestation in Early Modern Europe
Amy Eisen Cislo

3 The Prostitute's Body: Rewriting Prostitution in Victorian Britain
Nina Attwood

4 Old Age and Disease in Early Modern Medicine
Daniel Schäfer

5 The Life of Madame Necker: Sin, Redemption and the Parisian Salon
Sonja Boon

6 Stays and Body Image in London: The Staymaking Trade, 1680–1810
Lynn Sorge-English

7 Prostitution and Eighteenth-Century Culture: Sex, Commerce and Morality
Ann Lewis and Markman Ellis (eds)

8 The Aboriginal Male in the Enlightenment World
Shino Konishi

9 Anatomy and the Organization of Knowledge, 1500–1850
Matthew Landers and Brian Muñoz (eds)

10 Blake, Gender and Culture
Helen P. Bruder and Tristanne J. Connolly (eds)

11 Age and Identity in Eighteenth-Century England
Helen Yallop

Forthcoming Titles

British Masculinity and the YMCA, 1844–1914
Geoff Spurr

The Study of Anatomy in Britain, 1700–1900
Fiona Hutton

Interpreting Sexual Violence, 1660–1800
Anne Greenfield (ed.)

Women, Agency and the Law, 1300–1700
Bronach Kane and Fiona Williamson (eds)

Sex, Identity and Hermaphrodites in Iberia, 1500–1800
Richard Cleminson and Francisco Vázquez García

The English Execution Narrative, 1200–1700
Katherine Royer

THE POLITICS OF REPRODUCTION IN OTTOMAN SOCIETY, 1838–1900

BY

Gülhan Balsoy

Routledge
Taylor & Francis Group
LONDON AND NEW YORK

First published 2013 by Pickering & Chatto (Publishers) Limited

Published 2016 by Routledge
2 Park Square, Milton Park, Abingdon, Oxfordshire OX14 4RN
711 Third Avenue, New York, NY 10017, USA

First issued in paperback 2015

Routledge is an imprint of the Taylor & Francis Group, an informa business

BRITISH LIBRARY CATALOGUING IN PUBLICATION DATA

Balsoy, Gulhan.
The politics of reproduction in Ottoman society, 1838–1900. – (The body, gender and culture)
1. Turkey – Population policy – History – 19th century. 2. Human reproduction – Government policy – Turkey – History – 19th century. 3. Fertility, Human – Political aspects – Turkey – History – 19th century.
I. Title II. Series
304.6'6'09561'09034-dc23

ISBN-13: 978-1-138-66200-1 (pbk)
ISBN-13: 978-1-8489-3325-5 (hbk)
Typeset by Pickering & Chatto (Publishers) Limited

CONTENTS

To my parents Yıldız and Metin

ACKNOWLEDGEMENTS

This book is the outcome of a very long process that started with my going to Binghamton University for my PhD. It was structured in three different countries: the US, Turkey and Germany, and was possible thanks to the generosity of many individuals and institutions that supported me in different ways. First among them is my late advisor Donald Quataert. I will be indebted to him forever for his constant support throughout my graduate education and beyond. His inspiration, intellectual generosity, encouragement and great patience guided me in the long journey of the research and writing stages of this work. I wish he had lived to see the publication of this book. Rıfa'at Ali Abou-El-Haj has been a great mentor with his eye-opening questions, forcing me to thoroughly reconsider my ideas, and intellectual stimulation during my PhD study. Since then, he has always been available whenever I needed him. At Binghamton University I was also lucky to be the student of Jean Quataert who contributed significantly to my development as a historian of women and gender. She has played an important role in the very foundational formation of this work.

During the research and writing stages of this work I received the financial and moral support of several institutions. Archival research for this work was conducted under the auspices of the Research Centre for Anatolian Civilizations. I want to express my gratitude for the residential fellowship I received, and especially to my fellows at the centre with whom I shared the very early findings of my research. I am also indebted to the post-doc fellowship provided by 'Europe in the Middle East – The Middle East in Europe' (EUME) programme, thanks to which I had the chance to revise and edit my dissertation and turn it into a book manuscript. I thank my fellow colleagues for their constructive criticism which helped and encouraged me to improve the manuscript. I would also like to thank the staff of the library of Centre for Islamic Studies (ISAM) who provided a very accommodating environment to me for a very long time, first when I was writing my dissertation and then later when I was turning it into a book manuscript.

It would have been very difficult to complete this study without the support of my friends. I am indebted to Selim Karahasanoğlu, Nalan Turna, Nazan Maksudyan, Tuba Demirci and Betül Argıt for their help and friendship during the initial research and structure of this work. I particularly want to thank Başak Tuğ and Dilek Akyalçın who have been more than dear friends. Besides sharing the difficulties of working and writing, they always helped me to find my way whenever I felt lost. Our conversations were not only heartening but they contributed to the shaping of my ideas too. Zeynep Türkyılmaz has been a major support especially during my year in Berlin, not only with her fondness, but also with her sharp way of thinking. Burak Onaran read the dissertation version of this work thoroughly, and his comments have been very helpful with my revision. I also want to thank Seval Şahin, who brought many great pieces of Ottoman literature to my attention.

This monograph would never have been completed without the full and unconditional love of my family. My family, Mine Erkaya, Işıl, Oya, Serkan Ayman, Serpil, Yeliz, Tuna and Ahmet Balsoy have all supported me in their own ways. I am grateful to them. I owe my love for reading and for books to my parents Yıldız and Metin. It is thanks to their unconditional support and affection that I ever found the courage to go after my curiosities and interests. When I became a mother myself I understood more profoundly how great a luxury it is to be the child of such wonderful parents. It is to them that I dedicate this work.

My greatest gratitude is to Ali and Hüseyin, the two most important people in my life. Although we have very different interests and different approaches to many things including history, my continuous dialogue and discussions with Ali on literature, politics, history, and of course usually on nothing provides me with the biggest motivation and inspiration to continue my work. I thank him deeply. Finally, despite all the difficulties of raising a child and conducting research, each and every day since his birth I feel how lucky I am to have Hüseyin. His curiosity and imagination, never-ending questions and total lack of interest in my academic endeavours is the very joy of my life.

INTRODUCTION

This book examines the politicization of reproduction in the mid to late nineteenth-century Ottoman Empire. In a period marked by massive demographic changes that made the Ottoman state anxious about the fate of its population, female sexuality was increasingly subjected to medical and legal control. In this book, I investigate the ways this control shaped the female experience of pregnancy, childbirth and abortion. Through an examination of these three subject matters, I demonstrate that, in the late Ottoman history, reproduction was not a natural experience but instead a political subject.

I argue that the population policies of the nineteenth century were predominantly formulated through women's sexuality and the female body. Although I do not focus on the quantitative aspect of demographic changes, the demographic transformations and the pronatalist battle fought to compensate the loss of population constitute the immediate historical context of this book. Amidst a period of demographic turbulence brought about by territorial losses, migration movements and epidemics, the Ottoman ruling elites sought to eliminate those factors that reduced population and initiated policies to promote its further increase. To achieve these two complementary goals, the Ottoman government focused its attention on the fecundity of women, sought for ways to lower the high infant mortality rates and control the widespread occurrence of abortion, especially among the Muslim women of the empire.

Ottoman pronatalism was formulated through three registers: the medicalization of childbirth and the professionalization of midwifery; bans on abortion; and the medicalization of pregnancy and the discipline of the female body. In order to decrease maternal mortality rates, Ottoman medical and bureaucratic elites sought ways to improve the medical standards of childbirth in the second half of the nineteenth century. Transformation and enhancement of the practices of childbirth brought the education and licensing of midwives, who were the prime agents delivering women in the Ottoman society. Male midwives and obstetricians were also educated and trained first in Europe and then on Ottoman lands. The use of new medical technologies such as forceps, and the opening of a maternity hospital were some of the other means through which medical standards at childbirth were improved. Moreover, the functions, rights and responsibilities of the midwives and doctors, as well as the boundaries that demarcated their practices, were defined by numerous laws and regulations.

The policies and discourses to ban abortion were the second major approach of Ottoman pronatalism. While the Ottoman authorities were trying to implement policies to improve health standards at childbirth, they also sought ways to decrease abortions, which they saw as the main means of birth control among Muslim women of the empire and hence the main reason of the shrinking population. However, Ottoman authorities did more than complain about the practice of abortion and besides criminalizing it by legal measures, they developed social policies to discourage abortion, such as offering financial aid to families to raise children. An anti-abortion campaign which stretched over a few decades was carried out on discursive, legal and everyday policy levels. Examination of the anti-abortion campaign reveals that population policies of the nineteenth century were framed by gender and lead to the politicization of female sexuality. The pronatalist policies sometimes held women responsible for the relative low rate of population growth, sometimes asked them to bear and tend children for the well-being of the country, but always invoked assumptions about femininity and what the ideal woman was like. Giving birth was seen as a humanitarian and national duty, while abortion was associated with murder.

In the period I investigate, health care during pregnancy also received the attention of medical doctors. They maintained that a healthy pregnancy was the precondition of having a safe childbirth and raising healthy children. In order to draw wider attention to the importance of proper health care during gestation, they expressed their ideas by publishing advice books targeting pregnant women. The prescriptive literature on pregnancy conceptualized this important female experience as a medical event that should be checked and controlled by the experts. The normative sources redefined the female body as a maternal body, and they advocated disciplining this body in the light of prescriptions expressed by medical doctors. Along with the medicalization of pregnancy, the situation of those women who failed to conceive or experience pregnancy was also problematized. Female infertility was the final element of Ottoman pronatalism. Ottoman intellectuals and medical doctors saw infertility as the final factor hindering their goal to promote population increase and they sought ways to cure it through the latest medical innovations and the manipulation of diet and lifestyle changes. Through the examination of transformation of midwifery, bans on abortion, changes in the practices of childbirth, the medicalization of pregnancy as well as infertility, I demonstrate that Ottoman pronatalist battle was fought on medical, institutional, legal and discursive grounds alike.

The anxieties about the fate of the population were not universal, however. The government authorities were merely worried about the 'Muslim' population and overtly showed that they were not concerned about protecting the extant demographic composition. They lamented that while the Muslim population was declining, the non-Muslim, and especially the Christian population, was on the rise. In this sense, I challenge the idea that the Tanzimat ideals were about creating an 'Ottoman' identity formulated on the grounds of loyalty towards the Sultan.[1] I, on the contrary, argue that the concerns to create a more homogenous population started in the 1840s, much earlier than usually stated. The very basis of the Ottoman government's pronatalist assumptions was that the Christian population was enjoying growth and prosperity while the Muslim population was declining and falling into increasing poverty. The documents on abortion overtly express this idea. In this sense, this book significantly contributes to a rethinking of identity politics and the demographic prospects of the Ottoman government in the nineteenth century.

The history of the female body is one of the subtle themes of this work. Yet, I do not handle the concept of body in any direct way. The concept 'body' ties the subject matters of this research – childbirth, abortion, pregnancy and infertility – where the body seems most evident and most natural, yet political. The perception of the female body was not merely an outcome of natural processes, but was mediated through wider legal, institutional, medical, and discursive developments. The female body was a site of intervention on which the broader pronatalist policies were inscribed. In order to alleviate the anxieties about the demographic fate, the Ottoman state intervened with female bodies in direct and indirect ways. Through an empirical study of the changing practices of childbirth, the battle to control and ban abortion, and the medicalization of pregnancy and infertility, the ways in which the female body was lived, subjected to control and became the symbol of broader political transformations become overt.

The topic of this book falls interchangeably under the boundaries of the history of medicine and the history of Ottoman pronatalism. In its broader sense, however, this work is an attempt to gender nineteenth-century Ottoman history. Although the scholarship on this era is a rather sophisticated one, the transformation over this period is also recently being evaluated through the lens of women's history and gender analysis. Thus, one of the purposes of the present work is to fill this lacuna. Empirically, this research tries to unearth the experiences of women in Ottoman society when they were carrying children, giving birth to them, delivering babies or refusing to give birth for reasons of their own. Conceptually, it borrows the vocabulary and the analytical approach of gender theory. I am not merely interested in women, but I try to discuss the changing meanings of femininity in the Ottoman society.

There is not much novelty, however, in saying that the experience of pregnancy, childbirth, abortion and infertility are local. The understandings of bodily experiences are the consequences of their specific local and historical contexts.

Accordingly, one of the basic aims of this study is to show that even the seemingly most natural female bodily events are structured in diverse ways through time and space. Yet, the use of terms 'female bodily experience' or 'women' is not without problems since these terms may also totalize the experiences of a certain group of women over others. It is unfortunate that the scholarship on Ottoman history mostly has used the term 'women' synonymously for 'Muslim women' and overlooked the differences among Ottoman women along the lines of ethnicity, religion and class. In this work, although I avoided such generalizations, unfortunately I could not always adequately represent the diverse experiences of different women living in Ottoman society. One of the major reasons for this drawback is the nature of the sources which predominantly reflect the interest of the bureaucrats and medical men, and do not talk about women in direct ways. Nevertheless, my lesser attention to non-Muslim women of the empire is not because I find their experiences insignificant, but because of my failure to access sources produced by or about them.

Finally, the chronological focus of this research is bracketed between the 1840s and the 1880s. The first comprehensive law on abortion was issued in 1838 and in 1842 the School of Midwifery was opened. These two points in history demarcate expressively the attention the female body received from government authorities and medical men. Closing the bracket, however, was more difficult than opening it, since, rather than changes regarding the politics of female body, better achievement of the ideals that had been expressed for half a century marked the end of the century. In other words, I limited my attention to a period in which pronatalist anxieties were loudly expressed but not so successfully implemented.

Historical Context

The parameters of this work are cast by the broad and drastic changes of the 'long nineteenth century' of the Ottoman Empire. The topic on which this book focuses upon particularly falls under the purview of the Tanzimat reforms. Although recent scholarship emphasizes that the transformation of the functions of the state started much earlier by dislocating the announcement of the Gülhane Rescript in 1839 from the centre of historical analysis, there is a large agreement that this process laid a basis to redefine the state–society relationship by seeking to reconstitute the judicial system, eliminate the intermediaries between the sultan and Ottoman subjects, and heralding the principle of equality before the law regardless of faith or social status. Some recent works also argue that these changes permitted the emergence of public space as a ground for political debate and activity, despite its limited scope and the relatively low level of participation in it.[2] Although it did not receive much attention yet, issues related to female sexuality was as a topic of public discussion in this newly emerging political scene. Ottoman politicians, scientists, intellectuals, and medical doctors agreed that population was a crucial asset of national wealth and a precondition for prosperity and progress. They lamented, however, that, in comparison, the Muslim population was growing at much lower rates than the non-Muslim groups, especially the Christians of the empire. They, therefore, urged immediate legal, medical, and institutional measures and ushered in comprehensive policies that promoted higher rates of population increase and removed the reasons that hindered population growth.

The population was attracting mounting attention as a crucial national resource, while, at the same time, the Ottoman state was being deprived of drastic amounts of population due to territorial losses, nationalist rebellions and the formation of independent states, vast migration movements and epidemics.[3] Although the Ottomans enjoyed slightly increased birth rates in the nineteenth century as a result of enhanced health services, better sanitation conditions and increased infrastructure facilities, they suffered the loss of large territories which possessed high population densities including Greece, Serbia, Wallachia, Moldavia and Bulgaria.[4] The population, which was estimated to be somewhere between 25 and 32 million in 1800[5] was only a little more than 19 million in 1897.[6] The second half of the nineteenth century, moreover, was rife with major migration movements that further spurred populationist concerns. Close to 2 million Muslims fled from the Caucasus into the Ottoman Empire.[7] In this period, the Ottoman government also followed a policy to attract immigration into Ottoman lands.[8] The loss of territories that consisted predominantly of non-Muslim populations and the migration movements that brought Muslims to the empire significantly changed its demographic composition in the second half of the nineteenth century.

Perturbed by the rapid demographic transformation, and in accordance with the assumptions prevalent in European countries, the Ottoman statesmen and intellectuals associated the strength of the economy, the government and the military with the magnitude of the state's population.[9] According to the statesmen and intellectuals, demographic prospects were closely related to economic development, fiscal reorganization, administrative specialization and military renovation. Population was a crucial component of economic, military and fiscal power. Hence in order to regain an edge in the international competition, a larger population was needed.

One of the most crucial characteristics of the Ottoman demographic structure, however, was the low population density in large parts of the entire territory, notwithstanding significant variations between the regions. The major means of subsistence, agricultural production, was dependent on human labour. The land/labour ratio, moreover, was particularly low, which meant that large areas of fertile land remained uncultivated.[10] According to the Ottoman elites, the precondition for achieving agricultural growth was bringing additional land under cultivation, and that was dependent upon the supply of enough manpower for agriculture.[11] In other words, increasing economic activities in both agriculture and manufacturing was dependent upon the protection of the available population by maintaining its livelihood and security and promoting further population increase.[12]

However, the concern about population was not merely a matter of numbers, but its composition, control, regulation and surveillance were at the core of the new functions of the 'modern state'.[13] In the Ottoman context, starting with Mahmud II's rule, the relationship between state and society was increasingly defined in an array of mutual rights and responsibilities. The criminal code of 1840, land reform of 1858, juridical transformations, changes in legislation, bans on the slave trade, education, health and infrastructure services that were steadily provided to larger portions of the population and enhanced transportation and communication facilities, can all be envisaged as expressions of a modern sense of governmentality. As roads, railways, irrigation schemes, schools, hospitals, police stations and prisons were planned in accordance with population density, knowledge of the size, composition and mobility of the population acquired greater importance. These developments, moreover, presupposed a new notion of subjectivity[14] and reconceptualized population as a human 'resource'.

The extra funds needed to finance the new functions of the state, the establishment of education and health institutions, a modern army, infrastructure facilities and the enlargement of the bureaucracy, were, however, dependent on creating new means of revenues. Developing a wider and more efficient base of taxation and eliminating the intermediaries in the collection of taxes were two of the major means of generating additional funds.[15] The *tımar* system was abolished in 1830. Despite its significant limitations in practice, a more radical transformation was the transition to a direct and equitable system of taxation in 1839.[16] The new taxation practices, of course, did not simply subsume introducing new taxes and new counting methods,[17] but also demanded the enlargement of the tax base to include groups that had been previously exempt from taxation, which required enumerating and categorizing the subjects of the state.[18]

The pressing economic, administrative, fiscal and military needs required the mobilization of economic resources and human bodies. Its precondition, the urgent need for a sound registration system, was crystallized through the methods and premises of the censuses, as well as institutional changes. Although the majority of the scholarship on the history of population devoted its attention to the analysis of nineteenth century, the survey of land and human resources has a much longer history in the Ottoman Empire. The Ottoman state, from very early on, had quite an efficient system for counting its land and human resources and meticulously kept its records in *tahrir* (census) registers.[19] Such record-keeping was basically undertaken for the purposes of taxation and military requirements. In the nineteenth century, however, the Ottoman state sought new administrative responsibilities, in which knowledge of the empire's human and economic resources was necessary.[20] Censuses, land surveys and eventually a permanent population register system became essential for the government to efficiently maintain its functions.

Still, it is important to note that the first 'modern' census, begun in 1831, was not qualitatively very different than the previous *tahrir* registers. As Kemal Karpat also underlines, the raison d'etre of the Ottoman population counts at the beginning of nineteenth century was originally not the desire to have an accurate record of the total number of people within its borders, nor was it to gain hold of the details of the breakdown of the demographic composition. The main purpose, similar to the *tahrir*, was to establish a quantitative basis for the levying of personal taxes, and for the conscription of Muslim male adults into the army.[21] As such, the census was still not an end in itself in the 1830s. However, during the course of the nineteenth century, the changing nature and functions of the state, and the parallel reconceptualization of the population as a national resource, demanded new methods of counting. The novelty of the new census was not limited to methods, but included the motivation behind conducting them, which started to change as the Ottoman state broadened its interest from counting to controlling.[22]

In terms of institutional changes, the Office of Population Registers (Ceride-i Nüfus Nezareti) was established in 1830 and in only one year it undertook its first population census, which was completed in 1838.[23] With its large margin of error, this census was not significantly different than the previous methods of counting. In 1844, a second, but partial, census was conducted to survey the land and population resources in an effort to provide statistical information for the forthcoming reforms. The ways in which the concept of a functional government providing services to society were embraced, and how this affected the Ottoman census philosophy could be more concretely observed in the procedures, methods and approaches of the following census that started in 1866.[24] This census was conducted with the purpose of issuing to all Ottoman subjects an Ottoman identity card (*tezkere-i osmaniye*) and then to use it to register changes in the individual's status.[25] Hence the Ottoman state perceived counting in tandem with individuating, classifying and monitoring. In 1874, the Council of State (Şura-yı Devlet) re-evaluated the census system and refined the procedures for conducting the population censuses in order to establish a more concise and accurate registration system. Finally, in 1881, the council secured the establishment of a General Population Administration (Nüfus-u Umumi İdaresi) under the Ministry of the Interior (Dahiliye Nezareti).

It is significant that, as the government's census philosophy changed, so did the registration unit. In the traditional *tahrir* registers, the main unit of counting was the household (*hane*). For the 1831 census, the adult male, regardless of household status became the official unit. Finally, in the 1881 census the basic unit became the individual, regardless of age or sex.[26] Another significant indicator of the refinement of the methods of counting was the interest given to the registration of births and deaths. Until the nineteenth century, there was not any established routine of recording births, deaths and migrations. The earlier population registers (*vukuat defteri*), structured in the 1830s by the newly established Ceride-i Nüfus Nezareti, were virtually the perpetuation of the *tahrir* registers.[27] Through the course of the nineteenth century, registration of the population was handled in more diligent ways by identifying the drawbacks of the extant methods and pondering ways to improve them.[28] The census procedures to keep the population registers in local settings were also redefined in detail.[29] Although the problems were not abruptly and entirely solved, we can see continuous efforts to improve the procedures, to overcome the delays in registry and to increase the reliability and accuracy of the final records.[30]

In the main body of my research, I deal with the specificities of this broad picture in which population came to be perceived as a crucial asset of national wealth. I discuss the anxieties about the demographic prospects triggered by territorial losses, migration movements and epidemics. I focus on pronatalist policies that encroached upon the practice of midwifery, the experience of pregnancy and the decision to have an abortion. I handle these issues as a means to make the wider concerns about the quantity, composition and well-being of the population more meaningful. In this sense, I undertake a hitherto ignored task and evaluate the populationist policies, specifically, and the Tanzimat reforms, generally, from the perspective of women and gender.

Indeed, the history of the long nineteenth century is for the most part written in terms of institutional and legal transformations, which, unfortunately, remained ignorant of women and gender. The first serious academic works on women's history appeared in the 1990s,[31] and contributed in making women visible in Ottoman historiography. Unfortunately, other than a few articles published in edited volumes, the majority of the first generation of research did not employ gender as an analytical category of historical analysis, and the sex/gender distinction remained, to a large extent, unacknowledged. Still, it is very promising that historiography has become increasingly sophisticated in the last decades, and topics such as sexuality,[32] gendered aspects of law,[33] family,[34] education,[35] charity,[36] crime[37] and masculinity[38] are receiving due attention from historians. The increasing use of court records, moreover, helps to subtly reconstruct the everyday lives of Ottoman women and demonstrates the power structures within which gender relations were embedded.[39] This work also seeks to contribute to this literature by demonstrating the experiences of women and discussing gender relations in Ottoman society.

Sources

This research required a weaving together of sources produced by both state and non-state actors. The main body of the sources is from the Başbakanlık Osmanlı Arşivi (Prime Ministry Ottoman Archive) in Istanbul. I extensively researched and used ministerial documents, mainly, Dahiliye Nezareti, Maarif Nezareti and Zabtiye Nezareti collections, imperial decrees, and Meclis-i Vala and Şura-yı Devlet collections. I also used Dahiliye and Sıhhiye sub-collections of the Cevdet classification. While the imperial decrees helped me to systematically trace the regulations and governmental steps, documents from the Sadaret collection and the Meclis-i Vala were invaluable to have an idea about what was happening on the everyday level. Moreover, I searched several register collections, namely the Ayniyat registers and the incoming and outgoing documents of the Tıbbiye and the Sıhhiye registers. The Ayniyat registers consisted of summaries of the correspondence between the Grand Vizierate office, other governmental offices and local administrations. The Tıbbiye and the Sıhhiye registers also contained summaries of the incoming and outgoing documents of these administrations. Although these registers were very useful for delineating the daily functioning of these offices, it was not possible to obtain detailed information due to the brief and sometimes formulaic nature of the entries. I also did systematic research of the official codes and regulations related to broader medical issues. Finally, I tapped sources produced by non-state actors, specifically advice books written for pregnant women as well as normative and medical literature on infertility.

The nature of the archival sources as well as the specificities of this research made it extremely difficult to recover the voices of Ottoman women and their lived experiences. Due to the intimate nature of the topics that I discuss, it was almost impossible to find first-hand expressions of the experiences of women.[40] As I elaborate in the following chapters, the official documents that I based this research on offered only a partial view representing the interests of either the 'state' or the doctors. Neither the specific issues of this research – childbirth, abortion, pregnancy and infertility – nor its subtle theme – the changing perceptions of the female body – can be easily accessed through official documents. The government documents were produced in the context of the daily functioning of state offices, and hence reflect their interests and ideals. I also tried to overcome the bias of the documents by discussing them in detail with special emphasis on the context in which they were produced, their producers and their goals. Moreover, the assumptions about women, midwives and abortionists, which were inscribed in these documents, had specific ways of talking about the female body. It was these inscriptions and assumptions that I tried to uncover and translate into a meaningful story of the politicization of female sexuality.

I was lucky to find several dozen petitions written by midwives or ordinary people. The petitions, written by and about midwives, are mostly about their appointments, wages, leave, retirement and pensions. They illustrate the midwives' relationship with the government offices, their social conditions, needs and requests. As such, they offer us an otherwise unavailable image of their everyday practices and social and official interactions. The petitions written by ordinary people express their grievances concerning doctors and midwives. These petitions represented the difficulties they underwent when they became pregnant, had difficult births, or when they lost their infants.

Outline

In the first chapter, I evaluate the secondary literature on the history on midwifery and obstetrics produced from the 1930s on with a special emphasis on one of the pioneering obstetricians in the Ottoman Empire, Besim Ömer. Besim Ömer was one of the most prominent medical men of the nineteenth century with his contributions to the establishment of the first maternity hospital and enhancement of midwifery education. I argue that the modern historians working on the history of midwifery and obstetrics persistently took their arguments and approaches from Besim Ömer without contesting his facts or adding new ones. Whereas the histories on midwifery reproduced his scholarly production, the biographies on Besim Ömer reproduced his autobiographical accounts. Here I analyse the reasons for this identification with Besim Ömer and its impact on the scholarship.

The second chapter deals with the education, regulation and licensing of midwives. Raising the health standards at birth was crucial for decreasing the maternal and infant death rates. For this purpose, the Midwifery School was established in 1842 with the purpose of training midwives. For a long time, however, this education was not successful and rather than training, the Ottoman government devoted its attention to licensing and regulating midwives. I focus on the changes in the practices of midwifery and the reactions of Ottoman society to it.

During this period, pronatalist policies gained further visibility with the heating up of the debate concerned with limiting traditional birth control methods, abortion being the most controversial among them, which is the main topic of the third chapter. Although the government documents officially banning abortion initially justified this interdiction as a religious and moral obligation, as the different sectors of the Ottoman society entered the debate, the discourses on abortion were stripped of their moral and religious baggage, and the concerns about population were formulated on more concrete political and economic grounds. Here I argue that although the demographicist anxieties were formulated and expressed over women, this cannot be taken as a sign of absolute state dominance over female bodies, but the laws and regulations banning abortion, as well as the public debate on this issue, show that women not only gained legal subjectivity, but also became legitimate and legal actors of social change during this period, as part of the broader promises of the Tanzimat reforms.

In the fourth chapter, I focus on the medicalization of pregnancy and childbirth. Towards the end of the nineteenth century, the medical encroachment upon pregnancy and childbirth became overt. While the importance of having a doctor's check-up during pregnancy was highlighted, a maternity hospital was established for the first time on Ottoman lands. Although only the most desperate and poor women gave birth at this hospital and the women of better means preferred to give birth at their homes, the opening of such an institution mark the medicalization of childbirth. In the second half of the nineteenth century both medical treatises and advice books targeting pregnant women also started to emerge. In this chapter, I will focus on the advice books and discuss how they contributed to the medicalization of pregnancy.

Finally, in the last chapter, I deal with the ways infertility was redefined as a problem hindering pronatalist goals and how this turned into a public debate. While some of the Ottoman intellectuals saw it as a medical problem, others judged it as a punitive outcome of a wrongdoing. Accordingly, some proposed medical solutions whereas others recommended lifestyle changes and a more modest and moral routines to cure it. Yet, despite the differences of their approaches to the causes and cures of infertility, many Ottoman intellectuals agreed that infertility was detrimental to the real target of the family institution. According to them, producing offspring was a humanitarian and sacred duty and infertility was an important barrier hindering the economic progress of the country.

In sum, this work deals with the female experiences around reproduction that hitherto have remained unexamined to a large degree. It examined the ways pregnancy, childbirth, abortion and childlessness became the expressions of broader political contentions. In other words, it demonstrates how the intimate became highly political in the specific context of the nineteenth-century Ottoman past.

1 BESİM ÖMER AND WRITING THE HISTORY OF MIDWIFERY AND CHILDBIRTH

Besim Ömer was one of the pioneering obstetricians in the Ottoman Empire and ostensibly the most prominent among them for establishing the first maternity hospital and for improving midwifery education. He was born in 1862 in Istanbul, and in 1879 he started his professional training at the School of Medicine. After assisting Doctor Vahit, the instructor of midwifery in the same school, for a short period, in 1887 he went to Paris to specialize in obstetrics and *puériculture* (child care). In Paris he also followed the classes of Pierre-Constant Budin as well as Aldolphe Pinard. Pinard was at that time one of the pioneers of French eugenics, and his eugenicist ideas left a deep imprint on Besim Ömer's latter work as one of the leading figures of Ottoman and early republican pronatalism and eugenics.[1] Upon his return to Istanbul in November 1891, Besim Ömer started to teach midwifery and obstetrics to both the male students at the School of Medicine and the midwives at the Midwifery School.

In addition to his specialization in midwifery and obstetrics, Besim Ömer worked in other fields and published extensively, both in his field and on issues related to hygiene (*hıfzıssıhha*). Besides his achievements in enhancing midwifery education, he contributed largely to the formation of modern nursery education. Moreover, he was actively involved in philanthropic activities and took part in the formation of the Turkish Red Crescent, the Association to Fight Tuberculosis (Verem Savas Dernegi), and the Association to Protect Children (Himaye-i Etfal Cemiyeti). He wrote medical yearbooks, wrote and translated professional medical texts, published articles in popular journals and contributed chapters to medical collections. In addition to his scholarly work, he produced books on a rich variety of topics, including health care during pregnancy and infant care. Besides his medical treatise and the advice books about medical care, he had published four volumes of medical year books for the years between 1899 and 1906. Besides being one of the first people to write on the history of medicine, especially the history of obstetrics and childbirth, he was among the founders of the Turkish Society for the History of Medicine (Türk Tıp Tarihi Kurumu).

Thus, Besim Ömer was not only a prominent medical doctor, but was also one of the pioneers in the history of medicine.[2]

As one of the first male doctors to specialize in obstetrics, Besim Ömer was a major player in the history of midwifery and obstetrics, as well as Ottoman and early republican pronatalism. With his medical books and advice manuals, some of which were the first examples of their genre, he is a subject of historical inquiry. Moreover, because of his extensive publications on the history of medicine, Besim Ömer was a producer of history. For these three separate but overlapping positions, as an agent, a subject and a producer of history, a discussion of Besim Ömer's work, his account of the transformation of childbirth and the professionalization of midwifery, and his role in the formation of Ottoman pronatalism is important to this work. However, at the outset I should mention that this chapter is not a biographical account of Besim Ömer; instead it attempts to examine his imprint on the history of midwifery and obstetrics specifically, and on the history of medicine in general. Here, I will analyse Besim Ömer's impact on the later work on the history of midwifery and obstetrics. In other words, this chapter examines the impact of Besim Ömer on the scholarship of the history of childbirth, midwifery and obstetrics in order to encourage discussion of a certain structure of thought shared by several generations of doctors and historians of medicine in Turkey and the social uses generated by this historiography.

The choice to focus this chapter on Besim Ömer's influence on scholarship also offers the opportunity to pull together the four related issues that will be handled in this book: midwifery, abortion, pregnancy and infertility. Besim Ömer, with his multiple identities – an obstetrician and a teacher of obstetrics and midwifery, a devoted believer in pronatalism and a writer of pregnancy handbooks – has been both the actor of these topics and one of the producers of the discourses that redefined femininity and female sexuality. The discussion carried out in the present chapter, therefore, will also be guiding the following chapter.

In order to investigate Besim Ömer's impact, this chapter handles three partly overlapping bodies of literature and focuses first on the work of Besim Ömer himself, then the scholarship on the history of midwifery and obstetrics produced in Turkish from the 1930s on, and finally the first-hand accounts of the midwives, which are very rare primary sources. Based on these primary and secondary literatures, I will try to analyse a certain perspective shared by the historians of midwifery and childbirth and historians of medicine. Here, I argue that modern historians working on the history of midwifery and obstetrics persistently took their arguments and approaches from Besim Ömer without contesting his facts or adding new ones. Whereas the histories of midwifery largely reproduced his scholarly production, his biographies reiterated almost the same information about him. I argue that this repetition and reproduction indicates that twentieth-century historians continued to identify with Besim

Ömer, sharing similar motivations and interests regarding the place of physicians in the medical enterprise. Along these lines I will discuss how this situation shaped the writing of the medical history of the Ottoman society.[3]

'İhtiyar Acuze' (Old Crone) versus the Educated Doctor Saviour: The Work of Besim Ömer

Besim Ömer's work *Doğum Tarihi* (History of Birth), which later became foundational for the history of midwifery and obstetrics was published in 1932.[4] This small book is an extended version of the introductory chapter of the fourth volume of Besim Ömer's masterpiece, *Fenn-i Velade Külliyati* (Complete Book of Obstetrics). As opposed to this book, which was written for the students of medicine, the *Doğum Tarihi* targets a lay audience and it includes illustrations that were not used in the former treatise. As the subtitle, *Doğumu artırmak, ölümü azaltmak millî dileğimizdir* (It is our national desire to increase the childbirth rates and to decrease the death rates), makes clear, besides presenting the history of childbirth, this book also aims to advocate pronatalist ideas through raising the awareness of what constitutes a healthy delivery.

In *Doğum Tarihi*, Besim Ömer framed the history of obstetrics in three periods: the ancient period; the Middle Ages; and the modern era. His periodization became the conventional model of periodization for later work. The ancient period is characterized by the almost absolute control of women over childbirth. Besim Ömer, however, openly laments the exclusion of male doctors from labour and deliveries, mentioning that if they had been able to take part at childbirths earlier, they could have accelerated the progress in obstetrics at a much earlier date. During those dark years, in his words, midwives caused all kinds of harm to pregnant women and their infants.

Although Besim Ömer briefly mentions the practices of midwifery in ancient Israel, Egypt and India, his main emphasis is on the medical achievements in ancient Greece and Rome. Although this emphasis is partly related to the medical education he received in France, this choice hints at Besim Ömer's perceptions of the newly founded Turkish Republic. This choice is the outcome of an approach that tries to situate modern Turkey as a part of Europe and its science as distinguished from the backwardness of its Ottoman past.

The Middle Ages, according to Besim Ömer's periodization, started after the seventh century, and the role of Arabic intellectuals in medical progress was its epitome. According to Besim Ömer, since the presence of men during parturition was strictly forbidden in the Middle Ages, as it was in the ancient period, female control over midwifery survived. Because of this deplorable social tradition, these medical men could not contribute to obstetrics as much as they were able to do in the other branches of medicine. Nevertheless, Besim Ömer uncovers the contributions of several prominent medical men of the Middle Ages, such as Rhazez (Razi), Avicenna (İbn-i Sina) and Averroes (İbn-i Rüşd), who mentioned childbirth in their medical treatises. The emphasis on prominent medical persons has largely been shared by the later generations of historians of medicine. This approach evidently overlooks patient-centred histories, social practices related to medicine, as well as women and gender. And when patients, women and midwives come into the picture, they only serve to highlight Besim Ömer's judgements about their ignorance.

According to Besim Ömer, with the progress in surgery, the first caesarean operation and the training of midwives, the practice of midwifery started to change profoundly and the modern era in the history of childbirth began. Moreover, he shares the idea that it was the very introduction of forceps that characterized the beginning of modern midwifery and obstetrics. The use of forceps was a privilege reserved for male midwives and physicians; hence, this instrument symbolized the medicalization of childbirth in many historiographies.[5] Taken as such, one can see that between the lines, Besim Ömer had a strong perspective, deeply characterized by the notion of 'medicalization'. This term signifies the subjecting of a natural bodily condition, such as pregnancy, to the control and regulation of doctors and medical experts. This perspective is characterized by the emphasis given to the accomplishments of great doctors and significant medical developments, such as the introduction of forceps, the opening of maternity hospitals and the use of anaesthesia in parturition. This paradigm, however, has recently been widely criticized as I will explain in the following chapter.[6]

In *Doğum Tarihi*, while the history of midwifery was reduced to medical developments, the achievements of midwives or women healers were totally disregarded. Besim Ömer's strong tendency to conceive of the changes in midwifery through the lens of the medicalization paradigm, unfortunately, bequeathed a tradition to the scholarship which disregards the experiences of midwives, parturient women and the gendered practices of childbirth. As such Besim Ömer's account is a rather internalist one; he wrote the history of midwifery from the point of view of male obstetricians and male physicians, that is, his own point of view.[7] As a result, despite his claims to objectivity, his account is in fact highly subjective and presents the transformation of midwifery and childbirth through his own lens, as mediated by his own interests and through his own experiences.

The role of midwives in the long history of childbirth constitutes only a small part of *Doğum Tarihi*, and serves to express Besim Ömer's resentment of midwives' predominant control of labour and delivery throughout the centuries. In order to legitimize his point, this section of the book was supplemented with illustrations of midwives sitting on the women's bellies, or of them doing other atrocities to parturient women. His overriding aim was obviously to demarcate the scientific outlook of physicians from the superstitious practice of midwives.

With the exception of some French court midwives, this perspective palpably refers to the midwives in very negative terms. Besim Ömer appreciates French court midwives for letting physicians train them and going on to train other midwives, and for their fighting with the 'old crones' (*ihtiyar acuze*) even more than the physicians. However, according to Besim Ömer, other than a few such exceptions, the midwife was an ignorant, blabbermouth, filthy, old woman. Her single virtue was to jabber and prattle; she was superstitious and knew nothing about hygiene. Moreover, pregnant women, too, were ignorant and expected their midwives only to be sociable and amiable, rather than trained and professional. Like the midwife, they knew nothing about hygiene and believed only in superstitions. They very frequently paid with their own lives for their ignorance, which unfortunately was not a sufficient enough lesson to overcome it.[8]

Besides being highly subjective and essentialist, these views totally downplay the differences among women and their experiences of childbirth alike, across time and space. As also becomes clear from his praise of court midwives, Besim Ömer takes France as the model and tests the Ottoman case against it. His approach also establishes firmly the male physician/licensed midwife versus the old crone/ignorant woman dichotomy in the historiography of midwifery and childbirth. This oppositional pairing was indeed very common in the scholarship of the time, and it was first created in contemporary accounts, reinforced by state documents and then later by historians.

In a shorter piece published in the Medical Year Book of 1933, Besim Ömer once again laments that for many centuries not only the easy births, but the difficult ones as well, were monopolized by women, who assisted childbirths in 'primitive and treacherous' ways.[9] However, neither does he seem to be appreciative of the midwifery education provided in the School of Midwifery that started in 1842.[10] He points out that since the classes did not involve any practical training or involvement at childbirth, the education provided at this school was inadequate to raise midwives. He was also critical of the theoretical instruction provided at this school on the grounds that it did not make use of medical books, and that the students of the school, who were mostly illiterate, learned what their teacher told them by heart.[11] Besim Ömer also underlines the importance of maternity hospitals for midwifery education.[12] Although his point is very well taken, his only goal for drawing attention to this issue is not to argue for the establishment of the maternity hospital, but rather to criticize Sultan Abdülhamid II. According to Besim Ömer, for many years it was Abdülhamid who prevented the establishment of a maternity hospital because he was incapable of distinguishing such a 'beneficial institution' from a 'bastard house'.[13] However, I should remind readers at this point that the maternity hospital was in fact opened during the reign of Abdülhamid, and that Besim Ömer's assertion of Abdülhamid's ignorance was a political rather than a factual strategy.

Besim Ömer's later insistence on Abdülhamid's incapacity to understand the importance of a maternity hospital, and his hindrance of its establishment, has both personal and political reasons. It is known that Besim Ömer's father and brother were exiled by Abdülhamid; hence he had personal reasons to despise the sultan.[14] From a broader perspective, Besim Ömer belonged to a generation of nineteenth-century intellectuals who believed that Abdülhamid was a cruel despot hindering the progress of the Ottoman country. Like his coevals, he continued ever more fiercely to criticize Ottoman rule and especially Abdülhamid II, in the first decades of the Republic.[15]

As to his approach towards local midwives and ordinary women, Besim Ömer denotes them both as obstacles to the scientific progress of midwifery. It was emphasized that women, more often than not, preferred the old crones to licensed midwives. Those ignorant crones, according to Besim Ömer, dispersed many false lies and superstitions. They frequently used talismans, amulets and charms rather than medical methods during delivery, and these, he regretted, were appreciated by ignorant women.

Besim Ömer's perception of midwives and the ideal midwifery practice is overtly expressed in his pamphlet *Ebe Hanımlara Öğütlerim* (My Admonitions to Midwives). This pamphlet presents a rather full image of the midwifery practice in late nineteenth century and as such is an excellent source.[16] *Ebe Hanımlara Öğütlerim* includes forty admonitions to midwives and elaborately discusses pregnancy, labour and delivery, and newborn care. It demonstrates the medical procedures followed during parturition in the late nineteenth century. The ways to examine women before, during and after parturition, the tools and instruments needed and used, the precautions taken for safe delivery and the procedures to be followed during complications are elaborately described. This pamphlet, moreover, gives a comprehensive picture of the practices followed in the late nineteenth century by criticizing them and pursuing ideal alternative methods. In this sense, this manual is also an excellent source enabling a glimpse of late nineteenth-century medical procedures and approaches, as well as hinting at the mindset of contemporary doctors towards midwives.

This prescriptive book opens with Besim Ömer expressing his ideas and ideals related to midwifery. In parallel with his modernist vision, the pamphlet starts by drawing attention to the importance of education, training and hard work. Besim Ömer tells the midwives to treat rich and poor alike and to serve all women in need without discrimination. He also adds that midwives should be reserved and should not talk about the private affairs of the women they assist.[17]

One of the main issues brought forward in the pamphlet is the importance of hygiene and cleanliness. This pamphlet repetitively remarks on the filthiness of local midwives: their dirty hands and ignorance about hygiene. The strong association of the local midwives with filth and the doctors and educated midwives with cleanliness and hygiene is a very common stereotype that occurs not only in the medical history of the Ottoman Empire but also in the medical histories of other contexts. Besim Ömer similarly devotes substantial space to underlining the importance of hygiene. He describes the procedures for washing hands and for keeping the body clean thoroughly. He also draws attention to the importance of wearing clean clothes and the process of disinfecting clothes in case of exposure to a sick or dead body.[18] Furthermore, it is interesting that Besim Ömer tells the midwives to wear a clean, white, ironed coat over their dress.[19] The white coat metaphor is used as a symbol of medicalized childbirth. Although we do not have many images of midwives, the available ones demonstrate that midwives wore dresses according to their age, social position or economic sources, like women sharing similar social status. It was not the dress, but the ownership of midwifery baton and birth chair that signified being a midwife. Parallel to the demarcation between unlicensed local midwives and licensed midwives in the second half of the nineteenth century, a new measure was needed to distinguish the trained and licensed midwives from the ignorant ones, and the white coat served this purpose very well. In that schema, being filthy was identified with being evil; whereas cleanliness was equated with saving lives.

Moreover, in opposition to the midwives who, for centuries, were not only part of the shared female experience, but also an important agent of it, Besim Ömer believed that educated and licensed midwives should be outsiders who were supposed to teach women that childbirth was not a social event but rather a medical condition. Hence, she was told to forbid the practice of old traditions and to discourage visitors and the organization of ceremonies. Rather than being involved with such useless, even harmful activities, the midwife was supposed to introduce medical care such as regularly measuring and recording the temperature of the new mother and her room, and maintaining the cleanliness of the room.[20] Such new methods marked a new understanding of pregnancy and childbirth, within which the stages of the female life cycle were medicalized as well (for more on this, see Chapter 4).

While midwives were increasingly defined by reference to their medical tasks, the pamphlet makes clear that they were situated at the lowest echelon of the medical hierarchy. Doctors had the authority to examine midwives' hands or bags to see whether they were clean or not, and they could ask them questions to test their knowledge. Midwives, moreover, were reminded that they should call doctors in case of even the slightest medical condition, even if they believed that there was no need for a doctor's intervention.[21] The list of medical conditions that required midwives to call upon a doctor was very long. Considering that back in the nineteenth century, doctors also operated under relatively austere conditions and that they did not have much to do in cases of serious complications, I argue that these admonitions served to legitimize doctors' authority and maintain the medical hierarchy.

One topic that marks the boundaries between a doctor and a midwife is the use of medicine. Besim Ömer boldly asserts that midwives were not allowed to administer medicine to pregnant women or to infants. This, he notes, would be a violation of midwifery regulations even if the patient recovers upon taking the remedy, since such an act was considered a transgression of the boundaries of the profession as they were acting like a doctor.[22] Although midwives traditionally dispensed herbal remedies, the nineteenth- century ordinances and regulations banned them from doing so; midwives were only allowed to use or recommend some very basic remedies that were indispensable in carrying out their duties. Similarly, they were not allowed to use forceps, to undertake any kind of medical operation, or to turn the baby inside the uterus, although this latter procedure had been performed by the midwives for centuries. The prescription of medicine, the privilege to use new medical technologies and tasks that midwives had undertaken for many centuries, were now the prerogative of male pharmacists, surgeons and physicians.[23]

Finally, Besim Ömer reiterated that midwives were legally forbidden to perform abortions, he declared that midwives must not provide abortifacient drugs, or to help those who ask for an abortion.[24] As I will handle in Chapter 3, throughout the second half of the nineteenth century, the Ottoman government viewed abortion as one big social problem. This period witnessed a heated debate where young Muslim women were seen as the debauched agents of abortion and midwives as their accomplices. At certain times unlicensed midwives were regarded as the main culprits of abortion and were thusly condemned. In order to stop them from committing malevolence, their functions were strictly defined and they were banned from preparing abortifacient drugs.

The 'Angel Doctor': The Scholarship on the History of Childbirth and Besim Ömer's Impact

The Turkish Republic that was founded in 1923 rejected its Ottoman past in the 1920s and early 1930s, but starting from the mid-1930s Turkish historians began to show an interest in the Ottoman heritage of the Turkish Republic.[25] The change in attitudes towards the Ottoman past triggered an interest in the history of medicine, although it was more modest compared to some other fields. One of the earliest products of this interest was the emergence of the first Turkish journal on the history of medicine, *Tıp Tarihi Arkivi* (The Archive of History of Medicine), which was published by the Turkish Society for the History of Medicine starting from 1935. Many different topics related to the history of medicine were covered in this journal, and one of the first articles on the history of obstetrics was also published in it. This article was based on a presentation done in the United States by Doctor Saim Sağlık,[26] who studied in the Baltimore Carnegie Institute about women's hormones and was a specialist in women's diseases (*nisaiye*). Sağlık notes that he had benefited from the documents and personal anecdotes Doctor Refik Münir had provided to him. Refik Münir Keskingil (1881–1940) was, like Besim Ömer, one of the pioneering obstetricians in the Ottoman Empire. He taught midwifery at the Midwifery School between 1907 and 1912. After the foundation of the Republic, he held important governmental chairs: he was the president of the Medical Health department and the inspector general of the General Staff Health Services, where he retired.

This brief and highly descriptive portrayal of the history of obstetrics, like most of the subsequent scholarship, has a teleological approach to history, in which the Ottoman past is not handled with regard to its specificities but basically as part of 'Turkish' history.[27] One outstanding indicator of this approach is the portrayal of Avicenna (İbn-i Sina), who was indeed a Persian, as Turkish, and as one of the founders of Turkish medicine. It is not mere coincidence that Turkish historians, from the 1930s on, underlined that Avicenna's mother was Turkish, to claim that he was in fact Turkish.[28]

More scholarly work started to appear in the late 1960s. This work was, almost without exception, produced by medical doctors.[29] One of the examples that contributed largely to the formation of the canon is the work of Burhanettin Üstünel and Ertuğrul Bayırlı.[30] Üstünel was an obstetrician and the longest serving president of the major maternity hospital in Istanbul, the Zeynep Kamil Maternity and Children's Hospital. This cooperative account consists of three articles published as a series in the hospital's journal. The first part of this series focuses on the ancient traditions of birthing. The second part starts with a brief presentation of the Greek–Roman traditions of medicine, and then discusses the 'modernization' of obstetrics in Europe by putting a special emphasis on the developments in France. In the final part, Üstünel and Bayırlı present the history of obstetrics in the Ottoman Empire and the Turkish Republic. Similar to Besim Ömer's approach, this collection takes the European achievement as the model and measures the developments in Turkey against it. Given that the 'modernization paradigm' became the dominant approach in the production of history in the 1960s, the appearance of the Üstünel and Bayırlı article in this period and its subscription to that standpoint is not a mere coincidence. The linchpin of the 'modernization theory' is taking the state and bureaucratic elites as the main actors of historical change. This approach argues that the Ottoman state failed to modernize itself according to the European model and hence declined. This view neither conceptualizes the Ottoman Empire in a comparative perspective nor does it adequately address its specificities, but rather it tries to find the same path of development as in Western European contexts. Since this mindset takes modernization as the only goal, the histories written from such a perspective are only interested in the institutional steps towards it and the great men who enhanced these steps.

Along these lines and following Besim Ömer's scheme, Üstünel and Bayırlı organized their article in chronological order, in which antiquity, the Middle Ages and modern times follow one another. This type of periodization takes each period in history as a self-contained unit and fails to discuss the dialectics of change and continuity in time. Üstünel and Bayırlı, moreover, do not question how a certain period was distinguished from another, or what characterizes a certain period in history. As a result, all history is reduced to a succession of independent events and, accordingly, the single purpose of Ottoman medicine was seen as the preparation of modern medicine for the modern Republic. Finally, this perspective, takes the prominent medical men as the sole agents of the history of medicine, and either totally disregards women or associates them with superstition and malpractice.

A work that appeared only two years later distinguishes itself by tapping archival evidence and contemporary newspapers to investigate the history of midwifery education.[31] The scope of this work, produced by Nimet Taşkıran, who was also an obstetrician/gynecologist, is relatively brief and mainly draws on the initial phases of the midwifery education in the 1840s. Yet, the limited availability of archival evidence to researches in those years highlights its significance. Unfortunately, despite his contributions, Taşkıran did not escape from simply reproducing the ignorant, local midwife versus the saviour, doctor stereotype, maybe because of his standpoint as a doctor.

From the late 1980s, there have been several general surveys on the history of midwifery.[32] One significant commonality of these works is their production by medical doctors similar to the previous works. For example, Aykut Kazancıgil was, like his father Tevfik Remzi Kazancıgil an obstetrician/gynaecologist.[33] These works, moreover, reproduce the abovementioned problems related to developing a linear approach to history and failing to relate the rationale behind periodization. In other words, these works do not propose turning points in history according to major transformations, but first define the starting and ending dates of the periods according to broader political changes and then later delineate what happened in between. This mentality of periodization can also be extended to the larger volumes within which these articles appeared. For example, the proceedings book of the Congress on the History of Midwifery and Obstetrics, within which Ahmet Hulusi Koker's history is included, also comprises three articles on the history of midwifery which concentrate on the Middle Ages, the Ottoman Empire and the Turkish Republic, respectively. This division of labour according to chronological basis serves a political use and points out a certain conceptualization of the past, which tries to embolden the transformations brought by the foundation of the Turkish Republic and avoids acknowledging continuities between the Ottoman past and contemporary Turkey.

The second major issue – the silence on midwives – becomes overt as opposed to the loud appraisal of medical men as embodied in the personality of Besim Ömer. In the words of Ahmet Hulusi Köker, Besim Ömer was the 'Godfather' (*Ağababa*) of midwives, and midwives owe all they have today to him. Ahmet Hulusi Köker concludes with a question:

> It has been a hundred and fifty five years since the start of midwifery education at the School of Midwifery in 1842. Today, are there still women who deliver in the filthy hands of the ignorant crones who pretend to be midwives?

This whole piece, as well as this final question, once again brings forward the 'old crone' versus 'obstetrician/licensed midwife' dichotomy, which has been persistently counterfeited since Besim Ömer's first work.

This dichotomous opposition is also conspicuous in the biographies of Besim Ömer, in which he becomes the symbol of the superior characteristic of the male physician. Besim Ömer was identified as 'the founding father of obstetrics', 'the angel saver of women and children', 'hero of medicine' and 'the benefactor of Turkish women and children'. Some of the early studies related to him were produced by his colleagues, and their mission is limited to Besim Ömer's appraisal.[34] After the 1980s, with the rising interest in the history of medicine, Besim Ömer's biography once again started to attract the attention of historians.[35] However, rather than critically discussing Besim Ömer's place in the Ottoman and Turkish history of medicine, these works mystify him. In these biographies, midwifery education and the changes in midwifery practices before 1891, when Besim Ömer returned to Istanbul from Paris to teach obstetrics at the School of Medicine, were treated as practically non-existent or disdained.

Besim Ömer's texts have been foundational in two respects. First of all, almost all the later work based their accounts on his evidence and texts. The historians of medicine reiterated his information, framed their accounts in a similar model and, as a result, in the end, they reproduced the same approach. One outstanding aspect of the scholarship is the reference to the Greco-Roman tradition as the roots of modern obstetrics and midwifery, and the denotation of the Ottoman past in a very brief and usually demeaning manner. The midwives are also demeaned and their contribution is almost totally denied. According to the scholarship, the real turning point towards 'modern' medicine was characterized by the foundation of the Turkish Republic, and the Ottoman past is seen as an era of darkness, although the very same physicians, ironically, had their medical training in the Ottoman medical schools

The scholarship reproduces the dichotomy between the local midwife and the educated male physician and his assistant licensed midwife. According to this dichotomy, the local midwife is old, ignorant, untrained and superstitious. Her scant knowledge is based solely on practical experience and she appealed to traditions and magic in case of any problems. Moreover, she was mostly lacking in any feelings and was indifferent to the women and infants she murdered. The male physician, on the other hand, was young, educated, scientific and caring. He had a formal education and a theoretical understanding of female anatomy and the process of parturition. Hence, he was able to save the lives of women and infants, even in the most difficult conditions of birth. As opposed to the monstrous midwife, the physician was an angel and saviour.

These opposing characteristics were perpetuated and reinforced by some educated and licensed midwives as well. One of the very rare accounts produced by midwives, the short memoirs of the midwife Rasiha, *Resimli Ay* (1925), exemplifies this vividly.[36] In an interview titled 'What did I see in my twenty years of midwifery experience?', Rasiha tells of her experiences as a midwife. What she actually narrates, however, is the malpractice of local unlicensed midwives and their ignorance. Rasiha handles a number of issues related to pregnancy, childbirth and childcare and mentions some common mistakes that harm women and infants. She criticizes local beliefs, superstitions and bigotry, and recollects how these led to deaths. She had a very vivid style which was based on her personal experiences. In this account, ignorance is offered as the main cause of malpractice. According to Rasiha, unlicensed midwives were ignorant, knew nothing about the science of medicine and did not feel any necessity to train themselves. They were filthy and they had dirty hands, which they continuously wiped on their dirty dresses or even on the carpets in the houses they went. They, more often than not, caused the death of women and infants, and felt no guilt since they saw this as an outcome of fate rather than their own malpractice. It is also significant that whenever she encountered an atrocity of a local midwife, she did not intervene herself but rather called a doctor. As I shall expand on throughout the following chapter, although midwives were placed at the lowest echelon of the medical establishment of the nineteenth century, they were granted certain rights and benefits once they were licensed. In Rasiha's account, although there is considerable inequality of authority and power between doctors and licensed midwives, the latter are distinguished significantly from unlicensed local midwives. Both in practice and discourse, there is a considerable difference among the midwives. However, it was not only the material benefits granted to the licensed midwives, but the social and political roles that were assigned to them that constituted the basis of this difference. The purpose of these roles was to transmit a new perception of health and human life.

A similar approach to Rasiha's can be found in an interview with a midwife almost fifty years later in *Yeni İnci*, a popular women's journal published in the 1950s.[37] The midwife, Şahin, was also a former student of Besim Ömer.

This interview demonstrates just how vivid the unlicensed/ignorant midwife versus licensed/educated midwife dichotomy was, even in the imagination of midwives. Her memories are also framed within the licensed midwife/ignorant crone dichotomy. In many places throughout her interview, Şahin equates ignorance with local midwives and education with educated midwives. According to her, the licensed midwife saves lives; the ignorant crone causes death because of her false beliefs. The licensed midwife knows how to disinfect her hands and her tools, while the ignorant crone spreads infection with her filthy hands. The licensed midwife knows that she has to call a doctor in case of any complication, the ignorant crone is afraid of him because of her own faults. In short, it was not the doctor, but the unlicensed local midwives who were defined in opposition to the licensed midwife in Şahin's account, who also defined herself in opposition to the ignorant old crones. Şahin mentions that she was a student of Besim Ömer and underlines that she was to be a licensed midwife and not a crone, at the start. However, it is curious that here was a midwife who started midwifery via a very typical scheme; it is also significant that she delivered her first baby by chance when she had to attend a childbirth in her mother's absence due to illness, apparently before she was licensed. In many places she gives anecdotes of local midwives causing the death of women during parturition due to their ignorance and unwillingness to seek the help of doctors. Finally, at the end of the interview the journalist asks for any final remarks and recommendations for young women, to which Şahin asks them to avoid abortions. She says that giving birth will not deteriorate the body but on the contrary rejuvenate it. Even those last words demonstrate the links between modern midwifery and anti-abortion stance, which I will discuss further in the following chapters.

It is significant that Besim Ömer is not only used as the primary source of information on midwifery, but that his evidence and accounts are accepted as incontestable. Besim Ömer was one of the very benefactors of the newly established medical system, and he had an axe to grind when he was writing a certain type of history – one that virtually overlooked midwifery education that preceded his taking the chair of the Midwifery School in 1891. In other words, I argue that the cooperation between several generations of obstetrician-historians reflects a certain structure of thought which serves particular social and political purposes. The earlier generation of obstetrician-historians consisted of those who participated in the establishment of the new medical hierarchy, which subordinated midwives to the physicians. For the first generation of male obstetricians, one of the strategies used to gain social acceptance in a period when having male birth attendants was very rare and unconventional, as well as considered inappropriate in relation to societal norms, was to demean folk medicine embodied in the practice of local midwives. Especially in the second half of the nineteenth century, when the superiority of the practice of male obstetricians over that of midwives could only be justified with discourse, rather than medical practice, it was a common practice to argue that midwives were filthy, ignorant, old crones involved with superstitions rather than medical tasks, and that their work frequently led to fatal injuries. Later generations, too, sought to consolidate their increasingly accepted position both by consecrating the practices of their antecedents and blaspheming that of the midwives. Finally, the rare accounts available produced by midwives also mark out the divide between licensed and unlicensed midwives, and demonstrate that being within the same medical structure that promoted obstetricians, licensed midwives constructed their identities in opposition to the 'old crones', and not the doctors.

2 THE TRANSFORMATION OF MIDWIFERY

In 1853, the governor of Biga[1] sent a letter to the Upper Legislative Council (Meclis-i Vala) complaining that deaths during childbirth were caused by midwives in the town being neither trained nor sufficiently knowledgeable or skilled.[2] He appealed to the government in İstanbul for a suitable midwife from among the graduates of the School of Medicine to be sent to Biga, for a period of five to six months, to teach the science to practising midwives there, adding that the necessary expenses and allowances would be undertaken by the local population. Upon receiving the letter (*şukka*), the Meclis-i Vala contacted the head of the School of Medicine and asked them to appoint a midwife capable enough to teach midwifery in Biga. However, the school replied that although they had two midwives capable of teaching midwifery, these women were indispensable and could not be sent. After some further exchange, the governor of Biga was asked to choose one talented midwife practising in the town and to send her to İstanbul to attend midwifery classes at the Midwifery School. She would later return and train unlicensed midwives in Biga. The council, however, insisted that her expenses and allowances be covered by the town. Moreover, it recommended that the Biga governorate choose a midwife who had some acquaintances in İstanbul to offer her accommodation. I have been unable to trace the governor of Biga's response, or whether a midwife was able to go to Istanbul, or who she was. However, I know that this petition is in no way unique, and that it is possible to find many similar requests from other parts of Ottoman lands.[3]

Why then, were local governments asking for training for local midwives? How did this issue become a concern for them? We are lucky to have a case that was sent to the Meclis-i Vala, a few years after the petition from Biga, which can answer such questions to some extent. The petitioner, a certain Emine, who was an inhabitant of the Kemer village of the town of Edremit, in the present region of Balıkesir and a member of the Deziriler tribe, complained that her triplets lost their lives during birth because the midwife, known as the 'daughter of the fireman', did not cut their umbilical cords properly.[4] Emine requested the midwife to be put on trial and pay blood money. After receiving the petition, the Meclis-i Vala wrote an official letter to the governor of Karesi asking about the veracity of the event. The letter said that if there was any truth to these claims of malpractice such that the midwife had caused the death of 'those innocent ones', then it was a major misconduct. The letter also stipulated that the order to investigate the case had been given, adding that if the aforementioned midwife was really insolent enough to dare this misconduct she should be severely punished. However, despite the order of the council, apparently the case was not put on trial in the following year and a half, as evidenced by a second petition written by the same Emine.[5] This time, Emine briefly related the death of her babies, and then said that although she had presented the case to the governor of Karesi more than a year ago, she had not yet been notified about the conclusion. She also asked for a copy of the verdict. In reply to her petition, it was declared that the case had been communicated to the Meclis-i Vala, but no reply had been received from them. Of course the riddle is that the Meclis-i Vala did reply to the governor of Karesi, as evidenced by the document detailed above. Unfortunately, it is not possible, at least at this stage, to know whether the governor of Karesi did not receive the reply or received it but did not want to give it to Emine, or did not want to bring the midwife to trial.[6]

Yet, regardless of what happened to Emine, this case importantly offers us a glimpse of the local disputes and discomforts surrounded around the workings of customary health systems. In February 1867, for example, Hasan Efendi sent a petition to the school of medicine which stated that due to the malpractice of a midwife, his child had died and his wife had been crippled. He asked the school to revoke the midwife's license and ban her from practice.[7] In another case we see that a local doctor accused a certain Eftimya, who had been serving as a midwife in Adapazarı for twenty years, of causing deaths during childbirth. Although we do not know the details of her malpractice, we learn that provision of the wrong treatment was involved. Although the local doctor asked for her expulsion from Adapazarı, Eftimya did not wait for the decision without doing anything. She sent a petition to the Ministry of the Interior stating that she had a license and that she pledged to continue assisting births. The Ministry of the Interior finally decided to ban Eftimya from practice, but not to expel her on the grounds that she could be more easily monitored in Adapazarı, whereas she would more easily be able to assist births unlawfully in a place where she was unknown.[8]

Although the dominant discourses associate the deaths and injuries at childbirths with the 'ignorance' of unlicensed local midwives, reports of malpractice were in no way limited to them alone, but also involved cases both about licensed midwives and male obstetricians. In 1881, for example, the wife of a certain Kamil Ağa, who was one of the musicians of Ayakapı, started to have birth pains, but after hours of labour she still could not deliver. Kamil Ağa went from Küçük Mustafa Paşa to Cibali and found a certain Doctor Pavlaki there. Although the former asked for his help, adding that he would also pay the fee, the doctor said that he could not go to his house. Kamil Ağa immediately went to the local police, who tried to persuade the doctor to attend the birth. But when he adamantly refused, Kamil Ağa found another doctor with the help of the police, Malahiranos Efendi, who also turned him down. Finally, his third try was successful and Major Dalmatiko Efendi agreed to accompany him to his house and delivered the baby with a 'scientific' operation. Moreover, he refused to take the ten silver *mecidiye*s Kamil Ağa offered. After the birth and having his newborn infant safely in his lap, Kamil Ağa filed a petition to complain about the doctors Pavlaki and Malahiranos Efendi and to praise Major Dalmatiko Efendi. The Ministry of the Interior wrote to the Administration of Medicine (Cemiyet-i Tibbiye Nezareti) and asked that the two doctors be punished. The Administration of Medicine protected the two doctors from punishment on the grounds that Doctor Pavlaki had been very tired since he had just returned from a diphtheria operation, and Malahiranos Efendi was highly respected by the School of Medicine and should have a real excuse for his behaviour.[9] In another example, in June 1887, the infant Doctor Necip Bey was delivering died. Upon the complaint written by the father of the dead infant, the doctor was arrested and kept in custody for one and a half years, after which a petition was sent to the Ministry of Justice asking his forgiveness.[10] In March 1902, Doctor Manol of Yenice gave the wife of Andon Papa İstavri ergot to ease her labour pains, even though this drug had been forbidden. Unfortunately the poor women died and her husband placed a case against the doctor.[11]

Throughout the century, reports of malpractice cases steadily increased. I could offer further examples where ordinary Ottomans expressed their grievances about the doctors and the working of the medical system, if there were space.[12] However, it is hardly possible to conclude that malpractice itself increased; the increasing visibility should, rather, be searched within the broader pronatalist context where midwives were scrutinized and problematized by the populationist elites. As the Ottoman state directed increasing attention to its population as a source of national wealth, it turned its focus to midwives and their practice. Ottoman pronatalists believed that improving conditions at childbirth and decreasing the maternal and infant death rates were preconditions for achieving higher rates of population growth. This presumption led the medical elites to scrutinize the cases of maternal and infant deaths at childbirth, stillbirths and other risks during and after parturition. The assumptions about the high maternal death rates were, however, marked by prejudices held against traditional midwives; it was their malpractice and ignorance that was chiefly held responsible for high mortality at childbirth. Moreover, according to most of the medical elites, it was midwives who spread diseases and injured the newborn children. In order to fulfil the pronatalist goals, they surmised it was essential to first replace the traditional midwives with midwives educated by the Ottoman state, and then to monitor their activities. Accordingly, the second half of the nineteenth century saw the Ottoman state vigorously licensed, regulated and controlled midwifery. And although with the establishment of the Midwifery School the Ottoman state showed its aspiration to train midwives, its other, bigger concern was to render them completely under their control. The Ottoman state was caring about the health and safety of the pregnant women, but at the same time it sought to increase the population. For this reason, I argue, taking such a crucial female occupation under its control was closely related to broader pronatalist goals. However, as opposed to what happened in some other places, developments in obstetrics did not mean the displacement of midwives in the Ottoman Empire. Although the practice of male-midwives was becoming increasingly widespread in Ottoman society, this was not accompanied with the dislocation of midwives. On the contrary, in the Ottoman case, the real conflict was not between medical school trained obstetricians and midwives, but between licensed midwives and the unlicensed local ones.

Writing about the transformation of midwives' practices and the professionalization of midwifery is not an easy task, however, due to the relative lack of secondary literature available. Despite the wide attention the history of midwifery has received in other historiographies, this topic has largely been ignored by the scholarship on Ottoman history, in general, and Ottoman women's and gender history, in particular. The substantial body of the extant literature has been produced in Turkish, and unfortunately, scholars working in other languages have not shown adequate interest in this topic. It is also significant that this work has been produced mostly by obstetricians interested in the history of their medical branch, rather than professional historians. The extant literature predominantly consists of short articles, or the published texts of conference presentations, rather than full monographs. The reasons for these problems in the scholarship are manifold. The intimate nature of childbirth presumably led women to keep this experience to themselves. Moreover, it is true that most of the midwives, as well as the Ottoman women who were the prime agents of the debates on childbirth, were illiterate and hence did not leave much written evidence representing their perspective. For a long time, many historians presumed that there was no evidence on this topic and overlooked the documentation that was available. Finally, today gender history still remains at the margins of the scholarship on Ottoman history. This isolated image of the field discourages historians to do research related to women and gender with the apprehension that their work will not reach the appropriate audience. Admittedly this pattern started to change in the last two decades parallel to the wider developments in Ottoman historiography.

After the 1990s, with the increasing interest given to topics related to women and gender, midwives started to receive the attention of historians. Unfortunately, rather than in work concentrating mainly on midwives, we find them either in general accounts that try to depict the position of women in Ottoman society[13] or annexed to studies on Ottoman women in medicine.[14] The first body of literature, most of the time, over-generalizes disregarding the differences among Ottoman women along ethnic, religious and class lines. While the work produced by the second vein contributes to making midwifery a legitimate topic of historical research, it fails to acknowledge the power relations embedded in the conceptions of medicine.

The history of midwifery and obstetrics has been studied most extensively in England and for a later period, in the United States. Even in this relatively productive school, midwives have remained a mute group, and little attention has been paid to them, until recently. The contemporary accounts, which have a negative approach towards midwives and illustrate them as ignorant, filthy, aged crones serving a helpless female population, partly elucidates this ignorance.[15] It is very recently, and thanks to the developments in social history and women's history, that these accounts written by the founding fathers of obstetrics have been contextualized, and the medical disdain that masqueraded itself as historical fact has been uncovered. The early work of the feminist historians in the 1980s mostly concentrated on the biographies, work and experiences of individual midwives.[16] Although it is possible to learn a great deal about the midwifery practice and its links with local economy, politics, law and religion, when they are concentrating on the individual cases, this work occasionally tends to overlook the wider framework. One common observation about such earlier works is their focus on the decline of midwifery practice, and the midwife's loss of authority vis-à-vis the male obstetrician. Most of the time, these two points, the emphasis on individual midwives and their 'unmerited' decline, lead to a defensiveness and a romanticization of midwives as victims of developments in obstetrics.

After the 1980s, parallel to the debates and developments within women's and gender history, the interest in individual midwives gave way to an emphasis on gender relations. Instead of producing nostalgia for the bygone midwife, gender historians tried to understand the social control of birth and reproduction, the redefinition of maternity or pregnancy and the changing conceptions of femininity. To do this, they situated midwifery within a number of different frameworks, such as medical practice, women's work, gender relations or women's education. The use of sources such as regulations and licenses regarding midwifery, records of birth registration, censuses, court records, testimonies, pamphlets and literature on obstetrics have also added considerably to the reconstruction of the picture of early modern midwifery practice. As a result, the diversities of midwifery practices resulting from the urban/rural divide, as well as national differences and the impact of faith became more visible. The gendered approaches also problematized the Anglo-Saxon model, which was narrowed to the looser midwife and the state-sponsored obstetrician dichotomy.[17]

One of the major themes of the revisionist approach is the placement of midwives under a medical hierarchy through education, licensing and the institutionalization of public health.[18] Such work showed that, midwives were not merely victims, but they also enjoyed their newly earned social status in many ways.[19] Moreover, gender historians demonstrated that through an unofficial apprentice system, midwives were better trained than had been presumed, and their social and economic status were higher than had generally been accepted.[20] As the midwives' ignorance thesis had to be rejected, the causes of midwives' decline in certain national contexts became a question to be further dealt with.[21] Such work has also demonstrated that the relationships between medicine, state, society and gender cannot be scrutinized only through the professionalization framework, since this approach imposes twentieth-century standards to define professionalism.[22]

The challenge of the above model opened new venues to discuss midwifery. One of the topics that attracted attention was the disappearance of the 'social birth' experience with the medicalization of childbirth.[23] The 'social birth' approach argues that birth was a common and uniting experience for most women and that it constituted the core of women's domestic culture and female networks.[24] Gender historians demonstrated that as births started to take place, first with the assistance of male or female practitioners who were not part of the local female community, and then later shifted to hospitals, the practitioner rather than the parturient woman started to control the parturition process.[25] The medical technologies of birth;[26] the establishment of maternity hospitals;[27] the use of forceps, drugs and anaesthesia;[28] and medical concerns to diminish maternal mortality[29] are also scrutinized by women and gender historians. Finally, with the impact of 'linguistic turn', which is a term that marks the increasing emphasis on the analysis of discourses to understand historical change, gender historians examined the links between the developments in obstetrics and the changing definitions of femininity.[30]

Recently historians of the Middle East have produced rather sophisticated approaches towards the history of midwifery and obstetrics, especially in the Egyptian context. Mervat Hatem, for example, used the case of midwifery as an opportunity to question the discourses on modernity. Hatem argues that bequeathing a conservative social tradition, the newly established health and education institutions, including the School of Midwives that was established in 1832, in Egypt, did not contribute to the emancipation of women as the modernization paradigm concluded, but rather reproduced the existing gender hierarchies.[31] Khaled Fahmy, who similarly focuses on the School of Midwives in nineteenth-century Egypt, challenges the modernist view that contemporary observers of this school have commonly held. Relying on the school's documents, Fahmy asked a series of questions concerning its daily functioning, its impact on the students and the effect it had on society at large. Fahmy argues that the School of Midwives was not only a site of state control and surveillance, but also a terrain where the problems of modernization could be observed. Fahmy also rejects the dislocation thesis and demonstrates that it would not be fully correct to argue that midwives were victimized by state control. He argues that they enjoyed their newly earned positions. In other words, according to Fahmy, in many cases midwives both lost and won simultaneously: as state employees they lost most of their independence, but in exchange they gained protection from elite physicians, as well as from unlicensed practitioners.[32] Finally, the most recent works have an open emphasis on gender when investigating the experience of childbirth and the transformation of midwifery. Hibba Abugideiri investigates the role of gender in the British colonial takeover of Egyptian medicine at the turn of the century, and places midwifery within the broader medical developments, with reference to the construction of Egyptian womanhood.[33] Liat Kozma, on the other hand, approaches the changes in the practices of midwifery within the purview of legal reform in Egypt and its redefinition of women at the margins.[34] Both of these studies extensively exploit archival evidence and contextualize midwifery in relation to women and gender. I also seek to approach the transformation of midwifery in nineteenth-century Ottoman society from the viewpoint of women's history and gender analysis. I try to both present the stories of the individual midwives, whenever it is possible to recover their long-silenced voices, and to reflect upon the meanings of those stories within the broader institutional and medical changes.

The Establishment of the Midwifery School and the Regulation of Midwifery

One of the well-known accounts of Ottoman customs and lifestyles compiled in fourteen handwritten notebooks in the 1910s opens with a section titled, 'The Tasks Before and After the Birth of an Infant'. According to this detailed description, midwifery was a family profession, or a skill, like farming or childcare, that was passed on to succeeding generations without formal instruction and which could only be learned by experience. The midwife was not only a medical helper but also a handywoman. She met the expectant mother after the woman realized she was pregnant; checked on her once in a while; assessed the date of the birth; helped her to prepare the necessary items for the baby; attended the birth; stayed in the house to take care of the baby after delivery; helped the new mother with nursing; and treated any complications. In addition to her assistance during pregnancy and birth, she played a spiritual role. For example, a few weeks before parturition, the midwife would chase evil spirits away from the room where the delivery would take place using a slice of bread and a small amount of sugar put into a piece of fabric and then hung on one of the walls. Moreover, the midwife had an important place in the ceremonies after delivery: she swaddled the baby; named the baby; and celebrated the fortieth day after the birth.[35] After the delivery, in order to avoid childbed fever, the midwives also took care of the mother and the infant until the infant's umbilical cord was shed. Besides their medical assistance at childbirth, midwives were important mediators between women and the state through acting as witnesses or serving as experts in the courts, and inspecting women at the police stations when they were wounded, maimed or raped.[36] Because of their access to more intimate knowledge of women, the midwives played important roles within the female networks. In short, midwifery comprised more than assisting childbirths, and midwives fulfilled multiple social functions. Therefore, midwifery was one of the few profitable fields of wage work and career-making for women in the Ottoman society.

The transformation of midwifery practices started with the opening of the School of Medicine (Mekteb-i Tıbbiye) in 1839. Education at the school lasted for six years, with the fourth year including a course on obstetrics (Fenn-i Vilade), and the fifth year had a course on midwifery (Fenn-i Kıbale).[37] For use in the obstetrics courses, objects related to female anatomy, a female model with the skin peeled off, and models of the uterus and foetus at different stages of gestation were ordered from France in 1837.[38] Since the school did not admit female students, these classes were exclusively for male students. The Ottoman state's attempts to medicalize midwifery probably had limited results since the education lacked any practical training and there is no evidence that an average physician was better equipped, or more competent than the average midwife. Moreover, the number of male physicians who specialized in obstetrics did not quickly increase. In order to medicalize childbirth and provide enhanced health services that would diminish the maternal death rates, the Ottoman government had to find other solutions including training midwives and furnishing them with basic skills relating to childbirth.

The Ottoman governmental and medical elites had prejudices against the traditional, local midwives, and held them solely responsible for the high maternal death rates. According to them, midwives lacked scientific knowledge to deliver children without sever risks to mother and baby. One of the major contemporary newspapers, *Ceride-i Havadis*, which advocated the need for change in midwifery practices, wrote on its first page that childbirth was rife with vital risks, which were enhanced by midwives' mere reliance on experience. Midwives, according to the paper, ought to be trained and read books on midwifery, like doctors who, through the use of scientific books, were instructed in medicine at schools.[39] The newspaper also heralded that the mighty Ottoman Sultan who wanted the increase of the population of his subjects and the advancement of the welfare of his lands, was also worried about the difficult births of his subject women. In order to avoid the harms and pain during childbirth, the newspaper announces, the Ottoman Sultan appointed a French midwife, Madam Ventura, who first was trained in midwifery and then after adequate experience received her license.

Madam Ventura was supposed to help any Ottoman women, Muslim or non-Muslim alike, going through a difficult childbirth.[40]

As already mentioned, high maternal and infant mortality rates were intricately associated with the ignorance of midwives. According to Ottoman government authorities, during parturition, instead of taking the foetus out at once and cutting the umbilical cord, the midwives occupied themselves with superstitious things, hence causing the death of the infants.[41] The major means to stop these deaths was to gradually replace traditional midwives with ones educated by the state, which led the Ottoman government to open a Midwifery School in İstanbul in 1842.[42] According to their assumption, such an institution for the training of midwives would protect Ottoman women from the malpractice of traditional midwives, and gradually diminish deaths and injuries at childbirth as the number of the educated midwives increased. In comparison to the School of Midwives that was established in Egypt a decade earlier, in 1832, the Midwifery School in İstanbul did not comprise complete training in medical science, rather, its scope was limited to the instruction of midwifery and childbirth. The classes were offered twice a week for three to four months. One of the doctors of the School of Medicine taught the basics of midwifery science[43] in Turkish. After his courses, two midwives from Europe,[44] Madame Ventura and Madame Roberts, provided further training using models of pregnant women, pictures of embryos and foetuses from one month to nine months of development, and pictures and charts showing the various stages of labour and birth. They also taught about the possible complications that might arise during parturition.[45] Midwives who attended the courses at the Midwifery School received licenses at the end of the course. One major aim of the School was, eventually, to ban unlicensed midwives from practising.[46] Since the classes did not involve any practical involvement at births, it was barely possible to equip the midwives with better qualities than the local midwives who were already assisting births.

Despite the specialization of growing numbers of physicians in obstetrics, and the appeal of growing numbers of midwives to take licenses, the number of the educated doctors and midwives did not increase very rapidly, as the Ottoman government's sporadic attempts to summon unlicensed midwives to the Midwifery School demonstrate. Midwives were called to the school to learn the science, or sometimes just to take licenses with the implied intimidation that those without licenses would be banished from practice. For example in 1851, the office of the Grand Vizierate ordered the Marshal of the Police Force (Zabtiye Müşiri) to more carefully monitor unlicensed midwives.[47] Mentioning that many midwives evaded training and failed to take licenses, the Grand Vizierate lamented that maternal death rates remained very high. Additional announcements were made to midwives to come and participate in the formal training at the Midwifery School. Announcements were also made locally to ban unlicensed midwives from practice.[48] The numerous documents issued throughout the nineteenth century continued to associate the high maternal and infant death rates, the large number of stillbirths and the injuries during parturition, solely to the failure of the midwives to receive licenses.[49] The lack of data regarding education and the contrasting abundance of documents concerning licenses also lead me to conclude that, after a certain point, the Ottoman government altogether abandoned the goal to train midwives and limited its focus merely to licensing them. The preoccupation with licensing became overt towards the end of the century, and a remarkable indication of this attitude was the publication of the names of unlicensed midwives in local journals to denigrate them publicly.[50]

Besides the attempts to license midwives, the Ottoman government undertook steps to draw the boundaries of midwifery practice and demarcate midwives' tasks from those of doctors. One crucial component of this endeavour was forbidding midwives to use forceps and other obstetrical tools, reserving their use for male doctors with the formal Regulation Concerning the Practice of Local Medicine in Ottoman Lands (Memalik-i Mahruse-i Şahanede Tababet-i Belediyye İcrasına Dair Nizamname).[51] This regulation set the principles for the practice of doctors, midwives and pharmacists. Although the principles for doctors and pharmacists are further detailed and refined by subsequent regulations, the principles concerning midwives were left significantly rudimentary.[52] With this regulation, as previously mentioned, midwives were banned from turning the foetus inside the uterus; a task that they had probably been doing for centuries in the case of breech deliveries. Furthermore, procuring abortifacient drugs like *lolium temulentum* (bearded darnel) was outlawed with this regulation.

Finally, in 1883 the Council of State (Şura-yı Devlet) laid the still large number of uneducated and unlicensed midwives on the table with the aim of finding a permanent solution. By that time, however, it seems that education and licenses had turned into markers of privilege, since one of the issues handled in relation to licensing was the excessive fees male obstetricians and licensed midwives charged pregnant women who needed their assistance.[53] The Council accepted that due to these high fees, only affluent women could have 'scientific' conditions during parturition, while the great majority of Ottoman women were forced to seek the assistance of traditional local midwives, whom the Ottoman government adversely judged for causing deaths and injuries.

The precondition of the pronatalist policy to promote Ottoman women to bear a good many children provided better health services to increasing numbers of women. In order to encourage women to give birth to more children, the Ottoman government also started to offer financial aid to those families who had more than seven (and then later more than four) children and to those having twins or triplets.[54] As I will discuss in the next chapter, the government also tried to discourage abortion by legal regulations, as well as by a number of other social policies. However, in relation to its aspiration to diminish maternal and infant mortality rates by providing better health services to larger portions of the Ottoman population, there was still a long way to go. The establishment of a maternity hospital had to be postponed several times due to the lack of adequate funds, and the single hospital for women in Istanbul that offered lying-in facilities[55] was evidently insufficient for the population in the capital. In order to find a solution with limited financial sources, the Council of State decided that several doctors, who were experts in obstetrics,[56] could serve at deliveries in turn at the School of Medicine or at another suitable location for a reasonable fee.[57] Both the Municipality of Istanbul (Şehremaneti) and the directorate of the School of Medicine (Tabib Nezareti) were asked whether it was possible to find and appoint one specialist doctor to each municipal region (*belediye dairesi*) in Istanbul at a salary of five or six hundred *guruş*. Since this scheme would require a much lower amount, the Council believed it could be an alternative to a costly maternity hospital. Unfortunately, it became apparent that the salary offered was too low to hire expert physicians. Seeing the failure of this project, and pressed by the requirements of pronatalist policies and the insufficient funds to fulfil them, the Council faced the fact that hiring midwives was the only solution left, so they appointed four midwives at a salary of five to six hundred *guruş*. One of the midwives would serve in the Dersaadet region of the first municipality, the second in Kasımpaşa and environs and she would be responsible for the area from Besiktaş to Bebek in the sixth municipality. The third midwife would be hired for the Yeniköy municipality and would assist births in the area from Rumelihisarı to Büyükdere and Sarıyer, and finally the fourth midwife was hired in the Üsküdar municipality for the region from Kadıköy, to Üsküdar and Anadolu Kavağı. A doctor with a salary of one thousand *guruş* would also be appointed. He did not have a fixed location and was responsible for all the municipalities. In cases of difficult deliveries which midwives could not handle, he would be notified for help by telegram. Moreover, it was decided that those who could afford it would pay a reasonable fee but that the needy would be exempt from payment.[58]

In this period, rather than a radical shift, we see a gradual change of midwifery practices. Despite the desire to increase the number of male midwives and to license and regulate the activities of midwives, the Ottoman state was not always successful. The failure of education served to intensify the attention given to licensing. As a result of this failure, the Ottoman state tried to monitor the activities of midwives who were already practising through distributing licenses, defining the boundaries of their profession and establishing a medical hierarchy.

Regulations and their Shortcomings on the Everyday Level

Although the educational attempts seem to have failed for the most part in this period, the Ottoman government undertook crucial steps to license and to regulate local midwives and to bring them under its scrutiny and control. The increasing documentation related to licensing also demonstrates that ever larger numbers of midwives were licensed throughout the nineteenth century. In order to achieve this end, the School of Medicine and the Ministry of the Interior devoted considerable effort to structuring policies and defining the procedures for licensing midwives, doctors and pharmacists in Ottoman lands. Especially in the 1880s, however, the drawbacks of these official regulations became ubiquitous, as various contestations, questions and communications testify. After the promulgation of the 1881 regulation, the Ministry of the Interior sent a memorandum to the provincial governments[59] ordering that doctors, pharmacists, surgeons and midwives who lacked licenses issued by the School of Medicine should take exams at the premises of the school and then receive their licenses pending success in the examination.[60] While many provincial centres consented,[61] there were a considerable number of others who contested this direction. The governorate of Jerusalem, for example, mentioned that since there were a substantial number of doctors, pharmacists and midwives in the city who lacked licenses, their travel to Istanbul would create problems in the provision of medical services.[62] As a result, the governorate of Jerusalem asked the School of Medicine to establish a committee to examine doctors and pharmacists in that city. Protests were also raised in Bagdad. The Bagdad governor informed the head of the School of Medicine that not a single pharmacist in the city carried a license. He similarly argued that, owing to the shortages of medicine, a disaster might take place if the medical experts left the city to travel to the capital. The governor made the same proposal to the Jerusalem governor and asked the School of Medicine to send a committee to Bagdad in order to administer the exam locally.[63] Although the government at Istanbul and the Administration of Health (Sıhhiye Nezareti) did not support such solutions, the local authorities did not give up easily.

The presence of foreign doctors, pharmacists and midwives in provincial towns further complicated the debate. The Russian consulate in Jerusalem, for example, participated in the debate and communicated to Istanbul that, unless the embassy in Istanbul sent them a directive asking them to abide by the order, they would not comply.[64] This contest was soon followed by consulates of England and Austria in the same city.[65] The English consulate sent a note arguing that the new regulation was not fair and it discriminated against experienced medical staff by disregarding their services thus far, and put them in the same group at the newcomers. The consulate declared that the English doctors could not be forced to go to Istanbul to take the exam.[66]

Istanbul at first tried to stand fast and stated that the regulation could not be changed and those who failed to take the exam would be banished from practice within three months.[67] It also increased the tension by notifying the consulates that their embassies had no say, hence the contestations would not be taken into consideration. Moreover, Istanbul wrote once more to the governor of Jerusalem stating that doctors, pharmacists, surgeons and midwives could not perform medical tasks unless they were licensed by the School of Medicine. Finally, the embassies agreed to send the licenses of the medical personnel to Istanbul, and Istanbul finally accepted that it was not really practical for all the medical experts to travel to the capital.[68]

The procedure concerning foreign medical specialists was a topic of controversy not only between the consulates, provincial administrations and the government, but also among government offices in Istanbul. While the Ottoman state officials were trying to be resolute against the consular contestations, they were not actually very clear about the correct procedures, as their internal correspondence demonstrate. For example, after the contestation of the Russian embassy, several offices including the Ministry of the Interior, the Administration of Medicine (Tıbbiye Nezareti) and the Ministry of Foreign Affairs wrote to each other asking if the regulation concerned all foreign doctors, pharmacists and midwives no matter whether they had foreign licenses or not, or only those foreign ones without licenses.[69]

The status of the medical diplomas or licenses from foreign countries was also another topic of confusion.[70] It is noteworthy that it was again the provincial administrations which first realized the caveats of the procedures that the Istanbul government strove to establish. A document from the city of Kars first urged the government to clearly redefine the procedures regarding the medical staff that had foreign licenses. The Kars governorate wrote to the Ministry of the Interior and asked whether or not the four English doctors in the town who carried diplomas from the Faculty of Medicine in London also had to take licenses from the School of Medicine.[71] Faced with the shortcomings of the regulation, the Ministry of the Interior, the School of Medicine and the Administration of Medicine started a process to fill the gaps to avoid further contestations and complaints. The documentation of the correspondence between different government offices shows that none of those offices were sure about the appropriate procedure or the documents needed.[72] However, through a cooperative effort, the Ministry of the Interior and the Administration of Medicine tried to prepare information about foreign universities and medical schools including a list of their names, sample copies of their licenses and copies of their rules and regulations.[73]

The shortcomings of the regulation were not limited to the above issues. It was only later, and as result of the everyday difficulties, that the government offices came to discuss what was going to happen with the licenses of deceased doctors or midwives.[74] The rules and conditions concerning private doctors' offices was another problem that was recognized later.[75] In some cases, we can see that the Ottoman state was aware that the rules and regulations were still incomplete, but due to the urgent need for medical specialists some of the tasks could not be postponed.[76] Towards the end of the century, the problems on the ground also became more sophisticated and started to affect more people.[77] These, I argue, show that negotiations were not only taking place between the centre and the provinces but that the central government was also involved in a process of internal debate to determine the most feasible procedure that would not only consolidate its own power, but also help to carry out medical services smoothly and adequately. The regulations and policies were formulated with the participation of different government offices and followed intensive correspondence.[78]

Nefise Hanım and the Benefits of being Licensed

Can the intensive efforts of the ruling power and the medical establishment to license midwives be judged as the oppression of midwives? Although it is true that the nature of this important female occupation started to change in this period as a result of the government's pronatalist aspirations, the story is more complicated than the oppressed midwife versus the oppressor obstetrician dichotomy.

In July 1892, the governorate of Yemen informed the Ministry of the Interior that a midwife from Medina had passed away, and asked the ministry to send another licensed midwife to fill her position.[79] After communication with the School of Medicine in order to find a midwife who could travel to Medina and work there, the ministry made the decision to appoint Nefise Hanım to the town with a salary of five hundred *guruş*. Following the ordinary procedure, it announced that her salary and expenses for travel and resettlement to her new place would be paid locally from the municipal budget.[80] The ministry also informed the Umum Mekatib-i Askeriye-i Şahane Nezareti about her appointment.[81] However, Umum Mekatib-i Askeriye-i Şahane Nezareti informed the ministry that Nefise did not possess a proper license as issued by the School of Medicine, and hence her appointment could not proceed. Upon receiving this reply, the ministry wrote to the governorate of Yemen in July 1893 and informed them that Nefise could not be appointed.[82] The governorate of Yemen had its own plans, however, and immediately established a medical commission to examine her upon receiving this information. After the examination, the commission decided that she possessed the necessary qualifications to assist in childbirth.[83] The governorate of Yemen wrote a memorandum to the Ministry of the Interior and complained that since the former midwife Hafize Hanım's death, Yemen lacked a qualified licensed midwife. They added that the problem was exacerbated because Turkish women in Yemen would not accept Arab midwives to assist with their births. The governorate noted, moreover, that the majority of the available midwives found the five hundred *guruş* salary – which the municipal budget offered – too low and would not accept the position offered. Finally, attaching the report approving the proficiency of Nefise, the governorate asked for her to be appointed since it was very hard to find another midwife in such conditions.[84] The ministry was then faced with a real dilemma; the Yemen governorate's argument could not be easily overturned. Moreover, it persistently sent memorandums to impose its wish,[85] but the Umum Mekatib-i Askeriye-i Şahane insisted that her appointment was not possible according to Midwifery Regulation.[86] Finally, although the ministry ordered the Yemen governorate to search for another midwife, it was told to let Nefise continue to assist births until somebody else was found.[87] It was not much later that a licensed midwife was found. However, Ayse Hanım, the new midwife, asked for a salary of one thousand *guruş*, twice the amount that Nefise accepted. Neither the Yemen municipal budget nor the central budget could cover the extra salary. Ironically this financial controversy finally resulted in a solution in which both the Ministry of Interior and the Umum Mekatib-i Askeriye-i Şahane agreed that Nefise was proficient enough for midwifery and could be appointed to Medina.[88]

Nefise, it seems, was not fortunate enough, since she became sick in less than two years time after her appointment and wrote a petition to the Ministry of the Interior asking for permission to travel to Istanbul for medical treatment. She also wrote that, once she moved to Istanbul, she would not be able to return. Adding that she was completely alone with no one to take care of her, Nefise asked the government for retirement and a pension.[89] Now the Ministry of Interior first had to find another midwife for Medina[90] and then make a decision regarding Nefise's request.[91]

Nefise's story is telling. From the 1840s, increasing numbers of licensed midwives were appointed to hospitals in Ottoman towns and cities with fixed wages, regardless of their ethnicity or religion.[92] Although some could not be appointed to the positions they wished,[93] most of midwives were employed by the state. Being appointed by the Ottoman government secured them fixed salaries[94] funded mostly by local budgets.[95] Although these salaries were taxed by the government,[96] and it was not unexceptional that it was not paid regularly, having been granted this right enabled midwives to send petitions and pledge for payment of their due salaries.[97] Moreover, when they were fired, they sent petitions to be returned to their positions, and sometimes won their cases like the midwife Marya[98] or the midwife Inrit Roberts who managed to return to her position at the School of Medicine.[99] Moreover, being state employees granted them the right for a retirement pension[100] and protection by the government when they reached at a certain age.[101] When they died, their children could also receive financial aid from the government if they did not have any means themselves.[102] Additionally, midwives were awarded with medals for their services.[103]

Recognition received from the government made midwives important agents of Ottoman society. Receiving licenses and establishing a connection with the Ottoman government later permitted them to struggle for their rights. For example, a certain midwife, Muhsine Hanım, submitted a petition to the Ministry of the Interior stating that due to the increase of food prices she could not afford to live on her 1,000-*guruş* salary.[104] Muhsine asked the ministry to cover the rent of her house. The ministry forwarded her petition to the Council of State and asked for an investigation into her claims. The council not only decided that the salary was unsatisfactory, but also said that no other midwife should go to Basra and work there for so little money. It decided to increase her salary by 425 *guruş*, but did not accept her request for the payment of rent, since there were no similar examples. Apparently, the council was afraid that this case could become an exemplary case for other midwives, too.

While the Ottoman state was trying to control midwives and to set the norms of their practice, it was at the same time promoting those who were becoming part of the newly developing health system by offering them some rights and benefits. Although midwives were placed at the lowest echelons of the medical hierarchy, they were offered some advantages that unlicensed local midwives did not enjoy. Besides their financial demands, midwives also received additional benefits as state employees. They asked for leave when they became sick or wanted to visit their families.[105] They even asked the Ottoman government for help concerning issues not directly related to the practice of midwifery or medicine, such as the repair of their house when they did not have the money to do so by themselves.[106]

Moreover, in this period, the promotion of good behaviour was used as regularly as the punishment of malevolent behaviour. Midwives were sporadically awarded with medals, especially for their services at births. For example, in September 1891, the inhabitants of the Daye Hatun neighbourhood, close to Üsküdar, prepared a petition asking for the promotion of Besim Ömer and midwife Refiye who assisted the birth of Fatıma from the neighbourhood.[107]

The promotion of being licensed caused by the threat of banishment from practice as well as various benefits offered in exchange for taking licenses and being under medical and official regulation created a divide and conflict between licensed and unlicensed midwives. In this sense, in the Ottoman case, the conflict was not between the local midwives and physicians as in some other contexts. And it was the benefits offered to licensed midwives that formed the basis of this conflict, which can also be traced more vividly in the petitions written by the midwives. Take, for example, the case of midwife Kiryakice from the island of İstanköy (Kos) in the Aegean Sea.[108] The petitioner, midwife Kiryakice, stated that some women were assisting childbirths on the island without proper licenses. She said that the activities of these unlicensed midwives both risked the lives of expectant women and impeded her own means of subsistence. The petitioner also stated that she had submitted a previous petition to the local government, but that her solicitation was unduly ignored. This time she tried to gain the help of the central government. She first appealed to the local government, after seeing that it was not on her side she tried her chances with the higher authorities. It is also significant that what was at stake was not an ethical concern, but rather an economic one, which was expressed quite candidly in the petition.

Finally, in this period, licensed midwives were increasingly publicly recognized, a trend demonstrated by the advertisements and announcements in contemporary newspapers. It was quite common practice to announce the opening of midwives' offices in the newspapers. For example, *El Messeret*, a Ladino paper published in İzmir, announced in 1897, that a midwife[109] had just arrived in İzmir.[110] It conveyed that she would work at the municipality in the mornings, at the Osmaniye Pharmacy in Kemeraltı district in the afternoons and that she could be found at her house in the Bon Marche in the evenings. It is significant that the newspaper mentioned that her consultations would be free, which suggests that the municipality would pay her salary. Similarly, in March 1898, *Hanımlara Mahsus Gazete* announced that the midwife, Fehime Hanım, who was examined by the School of Medicine and awarded a license with a high degree, had accepted to be midwife for the journal. The journal announced to its readers that they could apply to the editorial office if they required the assistance of a midwife. Fehime would be informed from the headquarters and would go to the houses of those who needed her. The announcement mentioned that she had all the merits that a midwife should possess, such as tenderness, affection and mercy.[111] This shows that licensed midwives were becoming publicly visible, and that it was becoming increasingly legitimate to have them at births. Significantly, although her success in the examination was praised and her high degree highlighted, traits such as tenderness, affection and mercy were also emphasized.

Medicalization of Childbirth

In his vaudeville *Two Midwives and a Pregnant Woman*[112] published under the comic pseudonym 'Jüpon Bey' (Mr Petticoat), Mehmed Rauf, one of the most important authors of Ottoman literature, satirized a parturition scene. In it, a young pregnant woman, Behice, is divided between her traditional and superstitious mother, Hayriye Hanım, Western-style dandy husband, Raci Bey, and her father, Hüsnü Efendi, who satirizes both his wife and son-in-law's outlooks without a real belief in either. When Raci calls an Armenian midwife, Madam Annik, to deliver the baby, Behice's mother feels very uncomfortable with having the parturition with a non-Muslim midwife and believes that the birth will not go well and that the child will be villainous for not following tradition and having a Muslim midwife who would pray the formulas during delivery. Raci is not willing to stay in the house during the parturition and arranges a scene with Madam Annik, who sends him to her house to bring her toolbox which she has left at home. Aside, Madam Annik intends to call a male doctor so it is also for her own benefit that she sends Raci away. After checking Behice, Madam Annik informs the family that it will be a breech delivery, adding that this dangerous situation cannot be handled by a woman she asks Behice's parents to call a male midwife, Âli Bey. However, a misunderstanding occurs and instead of him, they bring Ali who is a specialist in haemorrhoids. After all kinds of funny and entertaining misunderstandings, finally the right doctor, Âli, arrives and delivers the baby safely. It is also significant that Âli is not an obstetrician but a medical student specializing in ophthalmology (*emraz-i ayniyye*). When finally Raci returns to his house and finds out that a male midwife has delivered his child, he becomes outraged, feeling that his honour has been tainted. However, Behice's mother and father protect the doctor who has safely delivered their grandchild.

Although it embodies the standard characteristics of its genre and taps into contemporary ethnic and sexist stereotypes for creating 'funny' scenes, this theatre play is significant as it demonstrates some of the views towards midwives at the beginning of the twentieth century. Having a non-Muslim midwife for a Muslim family was unconventional, and having a male midwife at parturition was definitely unusual, yet it was being accepted slowly by the society of the period.

In Ottoman society, childbirth was a female experience shared among women. See, for example, the well-known miniature image include below (see Figure 2.1).[113] This miniature depicts a childbirth scene where the parturient woman is accompanied by seven other women, a small girl and a midwife. The physical environment with wooden carvings and ornaments on the walls, the carpet with rich colours and patterns, the cradle, and the elegant birth chair, hint that the house belongs to a rather prosperous family. The women's clothing, including the new mother's, also confirms this. The women in the image all wear fancy dresses, some of them carry jewels, and they all have ostentatious headwear. The midwife, with her big headgear and fur shawl over her shoulders fits in with this affluent female atmosphere, and she probably shares more or less the same social standing with the other women. There is a serene and relaxed atmosphere in the room, as if it were not childbirth that brought them together but that they were simply enjoying each other's company. Two of the attendants hold the hands of the parturient woman, not to control her but to show their affection. The emerging of the infant announces that the most difficult and dangerous part of the delivery is over, and reinforces the sense of serenity and comfort. The presence of a small girl is also significant. Her neat dress and distance from the midwife suggests that she is probably not her assistant, but presumably the daughter of the parturient woman or of one of her companions. Although she is not helping at the time, her presence is crucial for future assistance. Through being raised among women and sharing those exclusive experiences she learns how to be a proper woman.

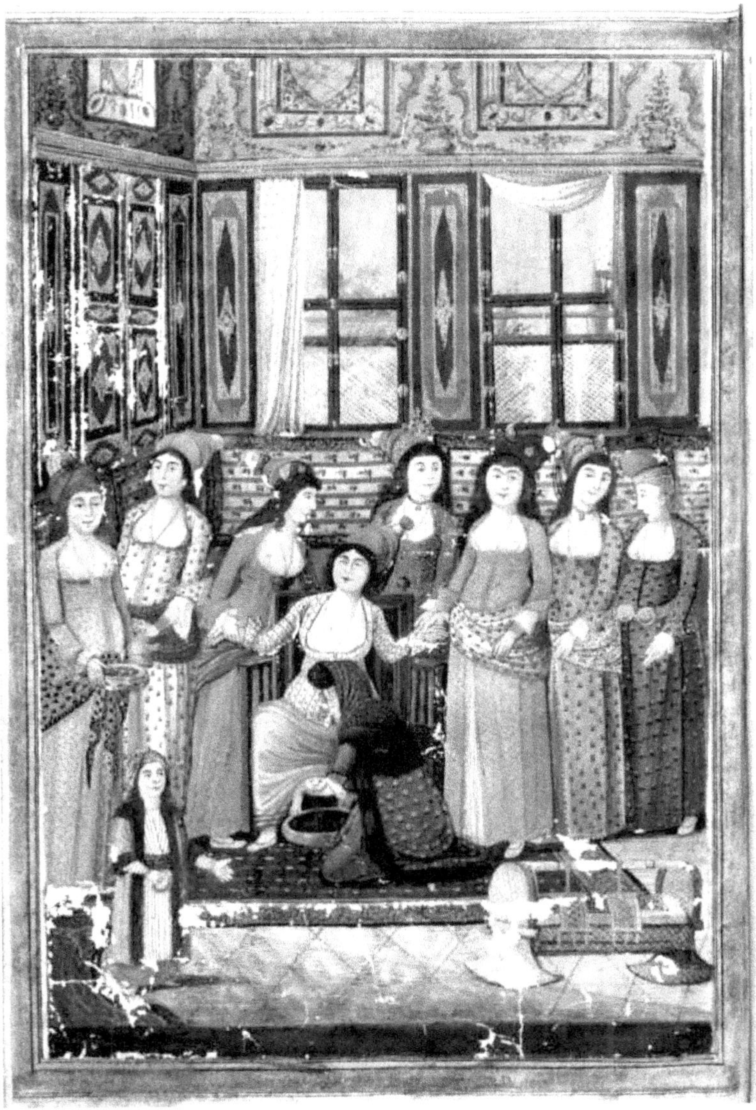

Figure 2.1: Childbirth in the Mansion (*Konakta Doğum*). Source: Enderuni Hüseyin Fazıl, *Zenanname*, Istanbul University Library, 5502 (1206 (1791/2)), 142a; reproduced with permission.

This image, produced in the eighteenth century, vividly illustrates childbirth being within the female domain and a shared experience among women. And this slowly started to change as midwifery became medicalized during the course of the second half of the nineteenth century.

At the mid-nineteenth century, Ottoman women still gave birth in their homes, and no private or state institutions existed for parturition. The first medical institution where women could receive assistance for childbirth outside their homes was the Haseki Women's Hospital, which was founded in 1847. The goal of the Haseki Hospital was not limited to providing health services to Ottoman women, but it was also established with the purpose of taking care of the lonely and destitute (*gureba ve fukara*) women of Istanbul. Apparently, at least according to the Ottoman government, there were many such women with no place to live and nobody to take care of them. Many of the most desperate women preferred to have abortions once they became pregnant, fearing that they would give birth on a street corner and fall into a miserable situation.[114] This institution provided assistance only to poor women, prostitutes and to those in the most desperate situations; married women with better means of subsistence could not imagine going there for childbirth. Yet its capacity was not enough to satisfy the demand. Hence, a maternity hospital, which would provide needy women with a healthier environment in which to give birth and which could also be used as an education institution, was, according to medical experts, an urgent need.

Two of the major goals behind the need to establish a maternity hospital were to train midwives and provide shelter for needy parturient women. Although providing practical training to male medical students was not initially expressed as one of the goals of the maternity clinic, towards the close of the century, as the limitations of instructing midwifery on only theoretical bases became overt, this issue was, also, expressed more vigorously. In that sense, the Ottoman case also fits with the approach suggesting there is a positive correlation between the maternity hospital and the rise of the male-midwifery and 'scientific' obstetrics.[115] Unfortunately, in the second half of the century, despite the ostensible goals, attempts to establish a maternity hospital failed until the first years of the twentieth century when it was finally opened.

In August 1869, after a meeting, the Council of State arrived at a decision to open a maternity clinic at Ahırkapı Otlukanbarı in order to provide both enhanced medical services to those women having difficult births and practical training in addition to theoretical instruction to midwives. The initial plan was to build a small edifice that had a ward, three classrooms, three rooms with a two or three bed capacity, one kitchen and a laundry room. The clinic was to provide lying-in facilities for eight to ten women at one time. After the approval of Sultan Abdülaziz, the Ministry of Finance was notified that the planned building would cost 145.259 *guruş* and was warned not to exceed this amount.[116]

Construction started a few months later,[117] and most of what we know after that, unfortunately, is limited to the payment of expenses. For example, in June 1872, the Ministry of the Interior ordered the payment of the due amount to cover the expenses.[118] Just a month later, in July, the School of Medicine wrote to the Ministry of Finance (Maliye) asking the ministry to tell the Treasury (Hazine) to pay the construction expenses that remained unpaid. However, in August of the same year, a huge change took place, and the Sublime Porte made a new decision that the building should be allocated to the Mekteb-i Tıbbiye-i Mülkiye Hospital with the construction of additional wards.[119] Despite its expressed need for a maternity clinic, the School of Medicine did not resist that decision, but on the contrary, sent the necessary plans, maps and financial documents to the Council of the Sublime Porte.[120] The Grand Vizierate also agreed to construct another additional building for administrative staff.[121] Moreover, it decided that the new building, constructed in Ahırkapı, would be used for educating medical students.[122] As a result, the original intention of building a maternity school at Ahırkapı was postponed, and the construction that had already started was transformed into the building for Mekteb-i Tıbbiye-i Mülkiye.

Two years later, in February 1875, the School of Medicine once again asked the Meclis-i Mahsus to consider the establishment of a midwifery hospital. It also asked whether the midwives could carry on childbirth operations at the Haseki Women's Hospital until an institution where they could receive practical training was opened.[123] The School of Medicine was told that in the short run, since it was not possible to build a maternity clinic, the midwives could be trained at the women's hospital on the condition that they be examined first to assess their competence in the practice of midwifery and in women's diseases.[124] In this period, we can also see attempts to built private maternity clinics that, unfortunately, failed.[125]

In 1885, the School of Medicine again asked for the construction of a midwifery hospital (Kabile Hastahanesi) in the capital, and this time the Sublime Porte consented. Now, the issue was taken more seriously, and even the architectural plans were commissioned. The architect, Perpinyani, drew the plans of a two-storey building with four wards for women in the post-partum period, two wards for pregnant women and three wards for quarantine in case of childbed fever epidemics.[126] We learn that several years later, the necessary funds still remained unpaid,[127] and unfortunately, despite the efforts made, this project, like the previous one, failed as well.[128]

After Besim Ömer returned from Paris to Istanbul, he started to teach obstetrics and midwifery at the School of Medicine in 1891. Probably due to the failure of those previous attempts to establish a maternity hospital, he opened a secret clinic in Demirkapı within the premises of the Topkapı Palace adjoined to the city wall in 1892. It was a rather small building, comprised of three rooms and a hall.[129] Despite its secrecy and small size, the clinic provided the first practical training in childbirth and women's diseases, with practice on living models and demonstrations of actual childbirth operations.[130]

Despite his secret work, Besim Ömer did not give up his prospects to open a legal and official maternity hospital. A document sent from the Ministry of the Interior to the Grand Vizierate's office, for example, demonstrates his imprint, although does not mention his name.[131] This document draws attention to the midwives' lack of scientific knowledge in childbirth, and the resulting problems and loss of lives during and after childbirth. In order to solve the problem, it was stated that a maternity clinic and a midwifery school had to be urgently established. In 1894, Besim Ömer sent a petition directly to Abdülhamid II. Mentioning that there were many maternity hospitals in Europe and none in Ottoman lands, he asked for the establishment of one in well-protected domains. Besim Ömer stated that this would cost two or three thousand *lira* at most, and he proposed that it be built in a predominantly Muslim district, such as the empty field across from the Şehzade Mosque.[132]

This request was treated positively and at last taken seriously.[133] The architectural plans were once again prepared, and it was decided that the hospital would contain twenty beds in three different types of wards. The third-class wards would be for commoners and cost twenty *guruş* daily. The second-class wards would have three beds and cost thirty *guruş* daily, and finally, the first-class wards would include private rooms and each cost forty *guruş* daily. The Şehremaneti (Istanbul Municipality) also tried to determine the price of childbirth operations (*ameliyat-ı viladiye-i cerrahiye*) but could not ascertain the fixed rates and concluded that the amount should be decided according to the income and financial power of the patients, as well as the fame and expertise of the doctors that would carry out the operation.[134]

The opening of the maternity hospital demonstrates the growing concerns related to a healthy pregnancy and parturition. While the clients of Haseki Women's Hospital were destitute women and the maternity clinic was notoriously known as the bastard house, we see that this final project was targeting provision of medicalized parturition and post-natal care to married and well-off women as well. In this period we also see the start of attempts to provide health services to pregnant women, or to those with small infants, as an important component of women's philanthropic activities. For instance, a play was staged at the Odeon Theatre in Beyoğlu district in 1908, and all its revenue was donated to poor pregnant women.[135] Along the same lines, many private maternity clinics were opened after the turn of the century by philanthropic women, in contrast to the examples that failed only a decade ago.[136] The Ottoman pronatalists also started to give increasing importance to the provision of medical services during pregnancy and childbirth, and the number of women who could benefit from these services steadily increased. A good indication of this situation is the extra food and drinks allowance provided to pregnant women and to women with small infants detained at the women's prison in Istanbul.[137] Moreover, pregnant women in prisons were also transferred to Hamidiye Hospital, where they could receive better care during and after parturition.[138] As previous discussed, giving awards such as medals or promotion to those who delivered healthy babies, despite the difficult birth positions, could be evaluated as another sign of encouraging more physicians to specialize in obstetrics.[139] Finally, I want to recall that enhanced health services were not limited to the pre-natal period, but were provided to women in the post-partum period as well. The medical measures taken to fight childbed fever epidemics also demonstrate that both Ottoman government authorities and medical doctors started to take childbirth more seriously.[140] At the same time, the authorities and doctors encouraged better care during the pre- and post-natal periods by persuading women to have more children, to avoid having abortions and providing enhanced medical conditions during childbirth through the education and licensing of midwives. In this period, one of the main means of accomplishing this was by advocating medical care during pregnancy through guidebooks that popularized the official discourses related to health.

In this chapter I have presented the attempts to restructure midwifery practice in Ottoman society through the education, regulation and licensing of midwives. I have shown that the Anglo-Saxon model that was based on the looser-midwife/state-sponsored male obstetrician dichotomy does not fit the Ottoman case. Yet, this does not mean that midwives were the ultimate winners, but that the picture was much more complex than standard historiography offers, and only through a gendered perspective could the complexities be adequately discussed. As the Ottoman state started to see population as one important source of national wealth, it could not leave the control of parturition to the ultimate monopoly of women. It tried to monitor the health standards at birth through its agents, the licensed midwives, and in return the Ottoman government offered them benefits they had not previously enjoyed.

The attempts to regulate midwifery can better be understood in the context of the establishment of a public health system. Midwives were situated at the lowest level of the medical hierarchy, and they were continuously exposed to the control of male physicians. They were not permitted to use the newly introduced obstetrical devices, or drugs and anaesthesia, or to perform more complicated medical operations, such as turning the foetus inside the uterus. Yet they did start to enjoy some newly introduced benefits. Moreover, their newly earned position, despite its inferiority to that of the physicians, allowed them to struggle for their rights and receive additional benefits.

3 ABORTION, POWER AND AGENCY

In May 1864, Sakratis, the pharmacist for the first battalion stationed at the Belgrade Fortress, was questioned about procuring abortifacient drugs for a Serbian woman, Isnato.[1] Sakratis was a graduate of the School of Medicine in Istanbul, and he had been working as the pharmacist of the fortress dispensary since arriving with his battalion five years earlier. Isnato was a thirty-five-year-old widow working as a servant. She had illicit sex with a Mösyö Lasiko Pirötin, a fur maker, and suspected that she had become pregnant. Mösyö Lasiko Pirötin consulted Sakratis, probably through his acquaintance with another fur maker that Sakratis had previously treated for syphilis, and asked for help. Sakratis went to the house where Isnato was working to check on her. Isnato complained that she had missed her periods for the last two months. According to Sakratis's testimony, Isnato looked quite healthy with red cheeks and she did not have any particular signs of pregnancy such as headache or nausea. Telling her that such complaints are very common among women, Sakratis gave Istano six pills that he had prepared, but did not check her chest or belly. He also told her to drink chamomile tea to ease her soreness. Two days later, Sakratis went to the house where Isnato was working to determine whether the pills had worked or not. It seems that they were quite efficient since Isnato had already had her period, though she suffered some pain. Sakratis told her to continue drinking chamomile tea until she felt completely relieved. After some brief bargaining, he took ten pieces of gold as payment from the fur maker, and that was the last time he saw either of them.[2]

Unfortunately, some four months later, and for reasons that we do not know, it was discovered that Sakratis had provided Isnato with abortifacient drugs. When interrogated, Isnato admitted that she had had an abortion with the pills Sakratis had given her. Sakratis was also interrogated for this misdemeanour,[3] and said that he had occasionally treated local people and, when needed, provided medicine for them that he sometimes took from the dispensary at the fortress and sometimes bought from the pharmacy in town. According to Sakratis, one day a fur maker had seen him on the street and, recognizing that he was a pharmacist, asked for help in healing his syphilis. Every day for a fortnight, Sakratis had gone to his house and gave the fur maker the medicine he had prepared.

Although he did not continue seeing him after the treatment, another fur maker, Mösyö Lasiko Pirötin, found him a while later, and took him to the house where Isnato was working as a servant.[4]

Despite a long and detailed interrogation, the local court could not make a decision, and wrote to the Principality of Serbia for counsel. The principality replied that procuring abortifacient drugs and inducing abortions was strictly banned by the laws. It asked the court at the Belgrade Fortress to investigate whether there was any evidence other than Isnato's own statement of not having her periods for two months. It demanded that the commission investigate whether Isnato had really aborted something and whether that had been analysed and identified as a foetus; whether Isnato took other remedies after the ones Sakratis had given her; and whether there was any other evidence. Despite Isnato's avowal and despite a few months' effort to investigate the case, the local court decided that Isnato had missed her periods for two months and that this was not enough time to know for sure if she was really pregnant. It also decided that the pills Sakratis had prepared were not strong enough to bring about an abortion. As a result, due to the lack of evidence, the commission concluded that Sakratis could not be condemned for procuring abortifacients. However, he was found guilty of curing local people and providing them with medicaments. Practising medicine without a doctor's license, as I explained in the previous chapter, was not tolerated in light of the regulations of the mid-nineteenth century. Sakratis was convicted of curing the sick without a doctor's license and hence violating the law.[5]

The case of Sakratis, the pharmacist, is quite unexceptional. The mid to late nineteenth century was a period rife with complaints about the ubiquity of abortion, and the absence of legal sanctions to discourage and punish the abortionist. During the time the Ottoman state was trying to improve the conditions of birth and diminish the maternal death rates by educating and licensing midwives, pronatalist policies gained further visibility with the intensifying of the debate concerned with limiting traditional birth control methods, abortion being the most controversial among them. The anxieties about depopulation turned into a public debate, and the otherwise conflicting parties of the Ottoman society agreed that abortion was the main reason for the decreasing 'Muslim' population, and hence concluded that it should be expunged. From 1838, various state institutions and ministries sporadically issued law codes and regulations to ban abortion and to punish those who practised it. Some of the Ottoman intellectuals, medical elites and men of science also participated in this debate and sought possible ways and means of preventing abortion. An anti-abortion campaign was launched, and while the government issued law codes, regulations and punishments, Ottoman intellectuals, medical elites and men of science showed support by expressing their anti-abortionist ideas through various genres including scientific articles and reports, literature and theatre plays alike.

The social history of abortion has attracted the attention of women and gender historians, as well as historians of medicine, and most of the time this topic lies between these two fields. Some gender historians, for example, have elaborated on the policies regarding abortion within the context of medicine, and have significantly contributed to demonstrating the inequalities inherent in the relationship between women and medical professionals.[6] The medicalization of the female body and the control of female reproductive functions has been another major focus of historians situating abortion within the context of medicine.[7] Discussing abortion in relation to women's legal and political agency has been another subtle framework.[8] However, most of the work on abortion, due to the nature of the topic and the lack of quantifiable materials, is faced with the constraint of dealing with the approaches towards abortion rather than the actual practices.[9]

In the specific context of Ottoman history, abortion has been most widely discussed with reference to its legal framework – either Islamic Law or nineteenth-century Ottoman laws and regulations.[10] The legalistic approach of the scholarship not only overlooks the complexities involved in the anti-abortion debate, but also almost totally disregards the main agents of abortion: Ottoman women. Moreover, the scholarship subscribes to an ahistorical perspective, presenting the approaches of the Islamic legal schools to abortion and Ottoman laws in a natural continuity without engaging in a critical discussion of the transformation of the legal approach and the procedures of justice. Such a perspective evidently assumes a succession characterized by an ideal unity – which virtually never existed – between and within these contexts.[11]

Nevertheless more recent scholarship has handled the history of abortion legislation through conceptual problems and tackled it in more refined ways. Selçuk Akşin Somel, for example, subtly discusses the unique place abortion occupies on the boundaries between Islamic Law and Tanzimat laws.[12] He argues that whereas some Islamic legal schools left more space for women to choose to give birth or to terminate her pregnancy, the modern Tanzimat reforms denied Ottoman women this freedom and exerted increased control over female bodies. Somel undertakes a compelling analysis and demonstrates that while the Tanzimat reforms were oppressive, they also contributed to the transformation of Ottoman women into legal agents. Tuba Demirci and Somel's collaborative work further develops this argument from a Foucauldian perspective and demonstrates the diversity of approaches towards abortion in Ottoman society.[13] More recently, abortion legislation in the Ottoman Empire and Turkey has received the attention of Ruth Miller.[14] Expanding on the fears of population decline, Miller subtly analyses the links between abortion legislation and citizenship formation. Engaging in a comparative analysis of three different contexts – the Ottoman Empire, Turkey and France – Miller argues that the criminalization of abortion was not only a signpost of the politicization of reproductive behaviour, but it was also indicative of the process of state formation.

Doing research on abortion presents several difficulties. First and foremost, abortion was – and is – an intimate issue that has almost always been kept secret or shared with only a few reliable friends or family members. As a result, finding first-hand accounts is extremely difficult and rare, and unfortunately, most of the available documents present the problem from the perspective of those who see abortion either as a crime or a serious misconduct. The medical treatises and other normative texts on abortion are limited to the analysis of discourses relating to abortion, and mostly fail to expand on the related practices. Moreover, they reflect the perspectives of the doctors who, sometimes, had reasons to exaggerate the problem. For example, in the Ottoman case, doctors attributed the entire scarcity of the Ottoman population to abortion without identifying other possible reasons. Overemphasizing this problem, presumably, enabled the doctors to challenge the activities of the midwives and to regulate, monitor and control them.

Along similar lines, work that handles abortion has to rely on documents such as court cases,[15] police reports,[16] medical treatises and other normative texts on abortion.[17] The bias of such documents, firstly, creates a fallacy that the society under the lens has many members prone to abortion. Secondly, in addition to the purposes for which they were produced, these types of documents solely present the stories of the most unprotected and vulnerable women. Since they had fewer resources to protect themselves, and fewer chances to find reliable doctors or midwives that they could turn to when needed, these women were more likely to come under police investigation than those who were married and more affluent. This situation led many historians to mistakenly conclude that married upper-class women did not resort so frequently to terminating their unwanted pregnancies. As a result of such problems, it is extremely difficult to reach relatively certain conclusions on questions such as who was seeking abortion, why did they seek it, what was their view of having an abortion, what were the means used, who were the professional helpers, what kind of networks did these women rely on, in what ways were the husbands involved and what were their views, and were the women having abortions mostly married women or those who became pregnant through illicit sex.

Unsurprisingly, my own research has suffered similar problems. Almost all the available documentation relating to abortion reflects the point of view of the Ottoman state and the medical elites. Considering the nature of the historical evidence available, it is difficult to conclude whether women really did resort to abortion more frequently than in the past, or whether the documents produced by the medical elites and top government bureaucrats exaggerated the problem for their own interests. The bias of the documents poses another problem, and in the few Ottoman cases available, I encountered almost entirely women who were widows, servants or whose husbands were imprisoned. Furthermore, the limited number of real case histories does not lend themselves to making generalizations and dense descriptions. Yet, as opposed to the official discourses emphasizing sexual lust and debauchery as the reasons for abortion, almost all the cases I was able to unearth involved cases related to poverty and vulnerability. Thus, as I will discuss further below, the attempt of the Ottoman ruling elites to construct a dichotomy between debauchery (*sefahat*) and misery (*sefalet*) as the two reasons leading women to abortion was a discursive strategy.

One such example, involving a doctor's examination in a case of suspected abortion, occurred in 1858, when Halise the daughter of Ahmet and the wife of Hasan Ağa had a miscarriage. Halise was a twenty-year-old woman living in the Haraccı Muihiddün neighbourhood of Sultan Mehmed village. After the miscarriage, a doctor Hasan checked Halise, together with a midwife called Fadime, in order to discover if she was trying to conceal an abortion. Halise had been almost six or seven months into her pregnancy, and she had the help of Fadime, who said that she had forcefully removed the foetus after she was sure it was dead. The doctor Hasan noted that the purplish marks on the head and body of the foetus was in accordance with the midwife's statement and demonstrated the force used. When the doctor touched Halise's belly, he found that her uterus and right ovary were swollen and badly aching. The midwife and the neighbouring women also told the doctor that Halise had lost a large amount of blood after she miscarried the foetus, and was still bleeding. Upon further questioning the women, in order to understand the reasons for the miscarriage, doctor Hasan learned that Halise's husband was in prison, and she went to visit him very frequently, despite the high temperatures of the month of August. The doctor concluded that it was too hot for a pregnant woman to move around, and as a result of her hard physical activity, her uterus had been infected. He noted in his report that Halise's case was not an intentional abortion but a miscarriage.[18]

Although the small sample of cases I have been able to unearth are not sufficient to propose a general model, it is not mere coincidence that all of them involved women who were vulnerable in some way. As I underline above, reaching conclusions about the reasons for abortion has significant drawbacks. Nevertheless, the very limited number of such cases does offer us the stories of women who tried to terminate their unwanted pregnancies. Rather than illuminating the reasons for abortion, such cases offer us the reasons for their documentation, which, I argue, is closely related to the change in perspective towards abortion.

Politicization of Female Sexuality: From Immorality to Illegality

This chapter analyses the Ottoman pronatalist policies targeted to ban abortion from the mid to late nineteenth century, and the reasons why Ottoman women so frequently tended to terminate their pregnancies, as explained by contemporaries; however, it would be misleading to argue that the discourses on abortion remained stable and fixed from 1838 to the end of the century. Until 1838, when the first ban on abortion was launched, the act of terminating pregnancy did not attract the attention of the government or the ruling power but was instead left to the religious domain. Until the mid-nineteenth century abortion fell under the purview of Islamic law, but there were different interpretations towards it. The absence of adequate terminology is significant. In Ottoman Turkish there were no separate words for abortion and miscarriage. The term *ıskat-ı cenin* was used to signify both of them. The term *ıskat* means to drop something, dropping the embryo or the foetus in this case.[19] Contemporary documents also use the term in both of its meanings. The specific meaning becomes clear only within the context in which the term was used. Causing miscarriage by physical assault, or by violent behaviour, has always been taken seriously and punished by Islamic law. In court records, accordingly, it is possible to find cases where somebody's violent act led to miscarriage, even in earlier periods.[20] *Iskat-ı cenin*, meaning abortion, did not attract the attention of the government or the ruling power but was left to the religious domain. However, in a society where there was more than one belief system, we cannot expect to locate one monolithic approach to the practice of abortion. Different belief systems had different approaches towards abortion, and hence Ottoman women of different faiths sought different practices. Moreover, the ways they justified or condemned themselves were also very different when they had to abort their children.

As I will argue below, the Ottoman elites did not try to ban abortion altogether in Ottoman lands; their main concern was preventing abortion among Muslim women of the society. However, even Islam and the law of Islam, Sharia, did not have one single fixed interpretation regarding abortion. More rigid schools of Islam either forbade abortion unconditionally or allowed it in the first forty days of conception and only when the mother's life was at stake. The liberal legal schools of Islam, including the Hanafi School (the standard legal interpretation in the Ottoman context), however, submitted that until the first 120 days of conception, before the foetus gained a soul, abortion was not *haram* (strictly forbidden), but *mekruh* (not forbidden but unwanted). Of course, the determination of the fortieth day and the period during which one can terminate the pregnancy without sinning was a topic of philosophical and rhetorical debate at a time when the knowledge of childbirth was limited and the mechanisms of fertility were not adequately known. Despite the diversity of their interpretations, the different legal schools of Islam have all shared the idea that since the mother is the origin of life, her life comes prior to that of the child, and therefore, abortion would be allowed if her life were endangered. However, the definition of the risks that justified an abortion was a major source of debate and demarcation among the different schools of Islamic law and their lawmakers. The Hanafi School, for example, again subscribed to quite a loose and liberal approach, concluding that becoming pregnant while nursing a baby, or the inability to breastfeed and the lack of financial means to hire a wet nurse were legitimate among other reasons.[21]

As the nature and functions of the state were changing, the Ottoman ruling power turned its gaze to the practice of abortion besides many other intimacies. In the last months of 1838, the Supreme Council for Judicial Ordinances (Meclis-i Vala-i Ahkam-ı Adliyye),[22] the Council of the Sublime Porte (Dar-Şura-yı Bab-ı Ali)[23] and the Council of Public Works (Meclis-i Umur-u Nafia)[24] exchanged ideas on abortion, the reasons for its ubiquity in Ottoman lands, and the possible means of preventing it. Although it is possible to find sporadic attempts to ban abortion before the nineteenth century,[25] this document issued in 1838, just before the announcement of the Tanzimat Edict, marks the upcoming of comprehensive policies concerning the practice of abortion.

In November 1838, the Council of Public Works produced a memorandum, both to express its ideas about abortion and to start a process to prevent its practice. The council stated that the mightiness and power of a country, its authority and magnificence, as well as its ability to continue the sultanate and to rule depended on the magnitude of its population.[26] For this reason, it was one of the government's primary duties to increase the population and to remove the factors that led to its decline. However, the Ottoman people, and especially women inhabiting Istanbul, were corrupted by the customary recourse to abortion. Clearly, this was the official start of the process associating depopulation with abortion.

The council presumed that there were two dominant reasons leading women to have abortions. As expressed by the council, some women had abortions because of self-indulgence and debauchery (*tenperverlik*), whereas others because of their financial inability to raise children. Hence, according to this assumption, some women, who avoided bearing children just to have comfortable lives, should be threatened and scared, while others should be financially supported to encourage them to keep their children. For the first type of women, the term *tenperver*, which evoked sexual lust, greed and avoidance of the burdens of childcare, was used. This type of woman tried to free themselves from the duties and responsibilities of motherhood, but yet did not abstain from sexual intercourse. In contrast, the debate on poverty referred to the family rather than women. When it was not women who were at stake, but the family as a social unit, the remedies, such as financial aid to ease the family's burden, were offered.[27]

Indeed, moral and religious themes occupied a prominent place within the context of those earlier anxieties about depopulation. The documents describing the harms of abortion and banning it used many different terms to denote abortion: abortion was against the will of God (*rıza-i bariye mügayır*); a shameful deed (*madde-i kabiha*); a mischievous custom (*adat-ı müstelzim-i muzırrat*); homicide (*katl-i nefs*); and a grave sin (*günah-ı azim*); and those who practised it would be subjected to eternal punishment (*mücazat-ı uhreviyyeye mazhar olacaklar*). It was both against the will of God (*irade-i Sübhaniyeye muhalif*) and caused the decline of the population (*tenakız-ı ahaliyi müstevcib*). With regard to the women who lost their lives while trying to terminate a pregnancy, these documents stated that death was what they deserved.[28]

However, when it came to defining the concrete means to discourage women, the Council of Public Works' main proposal was to order the chief physician to tell midwives, doctors and pharmacists not to procure abortifacient drugs for any woman. In addition, midwives were told to go to their religious leaders, the patriarch, rabbi or the chief magistrate, depending on their faith, and pledge oaths that they would not help women to terminate their pregnancies by any means.

In late 1838, the Council of the Sublime Porte placed the allegedly high level of abortion on its agenda and discussed it elaborately.[29] Emphasizing that other than midwives, doctors and pharmacists, many ordinary women knew how to induce abortions, the Sublime Porte stated that without controlling and disciplining lay abortionists, it would not be possible to conclusively remove the problem. One possible means of control, according to the Porte's memorandum, was to carry out medical investigations in reported cases of miscarriage to verify the cause. Presuming that neighbours would also be knowledgeable, the Sublime Porte then proposed punishing those who saw or heard of women having abortions and failed to inform the authorities. Finally, underscoring that the widespread occurrence of abortions in the provinces was a public problem, the Sublime Porte ordered that these decisions be published in the official newspaper, *Takvim-i Vekayi*, and distributed throughout the imperial territories.

Shortly after this initial correspondence, the Grand Vizierate wrote a memorandum to the chief magistrate in Istanbul informing him of the exchange of ideas between the three government offices regarding abortion, as well as the decisions reached.[30] The chief magistrate was asked to inform the magistrates of Eyüp, Galata and Üsküdar, as well as the chief physician, the patriarch and the chief rabbi about the oaths that midwives should pledge. Moreover, announcements were made throughout Ottoman lands regarding the upcoming measures to outlaw abortion.[31] According to the documents, since the prosperity of a country was dependent upon the magnitude of its population, avoiding unwanted acts that would decrease the population was not only meritorious, but also a religious duty that was to be rewarded by God. Yet, some people in Ottoman society were not afraid to terminate their pregnancies. Abortion was both against the will of God and the murder of the descendents of Adam.[32] It was homicide (*katl-i nefs*) and a grave sin (*günah-ı azim*), and those who committed this murderous act would be severely punished in the afterlife. Those who failed to thank God for having children would also be punished.

Despite this highly moralistic rhetoric and the emphasis on debauchery, morality and religion, the Ottoman government offices shunned punishing women in the initial stages of the process to outlaw abortion. While the documents persistently emphasized that women having abortions would be punished, either by death during abortion or later in the after world, they did not offer any concrete measures in this world. And in the limited number of cases where abortion became public and attracted the authorities' attention, it was the medical helper, rather than the women asking for help, who was punished.

Considering this approach, it is not surprising that the first criminal code promulgated on 3 May 1840,[33] only two years after the start of the anti-abortion campaign, included virtually no sanctions for those who performed abortions. An investigation of the criminal code demonstrates that neither the code of 1840, nor the amendments made in 1850, the 'New Law' (*Kanun-ı Cedid*), addressed abortion or defined any punishments for the crime of abortion.[34] From 1838 to the 1858, the single concrete measure to ban abortion remained asking doctors, pharmacists and midwives to pledge oaths against assisting a termination. Evidently no punishment was imposed to those who did not keep their oaths other than the threat of punishment in the afterlife. Although the documents openly resent the lack of punishment for abortionists, no amendments were made. Moreover, despite the ostensibly resolute tone of the Ottoman ruling offices that discussed abortion, and the numerous orders made to the chief magistrate in Istanbul, practising abortion remained practically legitimate until 1858, when the criminal code was rewritten.[35]

The case of a midwife called Mezalto is significant here. From a document dated 1850, we learn that Mezalto was found guilty of helping a black female slave who belonged to Latif, the master slave trader, to have an abortion when she was two-and-a-half-months pregnant, and she was banished to Salonika. Whatever the reasons were that raised suspicions against her, she was not condemned without evidence but upon the deposition of the chief physician, and after an investigation. Mezalto was an experienced midwife who had been assisting births for almost thirty years. After a year in exile, her six children sent a petition to the Upper Legislative Council (Meclis-i Vala) pledging her punishment to be discharged since she was too old and was in misery in Salonika.[36] Although we do not know the reply of the Upper Legislative Council, it is significant that the only conviction in this case was Mezalto, not Latif or his female slave. Moreover, this case reminds us that the absence of legal sanctions did not always mean the absence of punishment.

The 1858 code was the first to cover abortion under its purview and define sanctions against it. Abortion was covered under the broader chapter called, 'Abortion/Miscarriage, Sale of Falsified Drinks and Toxic Substances without Demanding Guarantor' (*Iskat-ı Cenin ve Karışık Meşrubat ve Kefilsiz Semmiyat Füruhat Edenlerin Mücazat-ı Mürettibesi*).[37] The first two articles of the chapter, 192 and 193, were about miscarriage and abortion respectively, and the remaining three articles were about practising medicine or pharmacy without a proper license and selling toxic substances.[38] Article 192 stated that causing a miscarriage by physical assault, or through any other means, would be punished by paying blood money (*diyet*). If the act had been done intentionally to cause an abortion, the culprit would be sentenced to forced labour, in addition to paying blood money. The next article, article 193, stated that any persons assisting an abortion by giving an abortifacient grug would be sentenced to six months to two years of imprisonment regardless of the pregnant women's consent. If the one assisting the abortion was a physician, surgeon, or pharmacist he would be sentenced to forced labour.

The 1858 criminal code maintained the approach that avoided punishing women who terminated their pregnancies, rather it defined sanctions against those who provided the necessary means and assisted in performing them. In addition, the boundaries between abortion and miscarriage continued to be blurred due to the double meaning of the term *ıskat-ı cenin*. Moreover, handling abortion together with other issues related to health in the 1858 code shows that by that time abortion was being stripped of its moral and religious baggage, and gradually turned into a profane matter situated within the larger context of public health.

The reluctance to punish women was a direct outcome of pronatalist goals that were dependent, in the first place, on women who were to bear the children needed to increase the population. Although the increased attention that the Ottoman government gave to abortion is a strong indication of the politicization of reproduction, it was not the women of reproductive age who were criminalized, but rather the doctors, pharmacists and especially the midwives. Of course, from the perspective of the Ottoman government, punishing women by any means, imprisonment, banishment or forced labour, would evidently destroy, or at best decrease, their reproductive capacities. The government needed female bodies to procreate the Ottoman population; hence, as a result, it shunned ruining the reproductive body by punishment.

From the late 1850s onwards, as anti-abortion bureaucrats increasingly associated abortion with poverty rather than immorality, a discursive shift also took place and the emphasis on morality was eventually replaced with an emphasis on material conditions. In other words, instead of debauchery, the parties opposing abortion came in time to emphasize poverty. They faced the fact that scaring women with otherworldly punishments was neither a sufficient nor efficient means of preventing abortion. Since poverty was the main reason for terminating pregnancy, financial aid was offered to women to encourage them to give birth. Accordingly, rather than using a normative language meant to improve the morals of women, or scare them with a religious terminology about sins and punishment, they appropriated a more neutral language to formulate remedies to encourage women to give birth to children, rather than abort them.

This change in the assumptions about the reasons for abortion also triggered a search for solutions. Along with the official government policies, some anti-abortionist medical elites also attempted to come up with solutions of their own to the problem of abortion, and only one year after the appearance of abortion in the criminal code, and the major organization of doctors in the Ottoman society, the Doctor's Association (Cemiyet-i Tıbbiye-i Şahane)[39] presented a report concerning abortion to the Grand Vizierate on 1 May 1859.[40] This report shows that the Doctor's Association considered itself responsible for the supervision of health in the Ottoman society and that it also explicitly shared the idea that population was a crucial national asset. Accordingly, it identified abortion as the major factor leading to depopulation and the consequent detrimental effects on international competition for prosperity. According to its report, the widespread occurrence of abortion was caused, on the one hand, by the lack of punishment for those who murderously terminated their pregnancies, and on the other, by poverty.[41]

The Doctor's Association lamented that abortion was considered quite legitimate in Ottoman society and that it was not secretly but openly practised regardless of class, in all echelons of society. When a woman decided to have an abortion, the time, the place and the means were not kept secret from others. The report told of the existence of specific locations that were publicly and freely used to terminate unwanted pregnancies without any uneasiness or shame. It also highlighted and criticized the lack of convictions, despite the presence of a code of law against abortion. Notwithstanding the implausibility of the first part of the argument due to the nature of abortion, the report also demonstrates discontent with the failure to punish the abortionist. The Doctor's Association argued that the 1858 law, too, would become void if it was not used, and proposed the establishment of a government office that would impose the law and punish the guilty. Only by putting the law into practice would women be discouraged from having abortions and the manners and morals of the population be improved.

The Doctor's Association duly devoted most of the report to discussing and finding remedies for the causes of abortion. Acknowledging that poverty and neediness were the two major reasons for resorting to abortion, the report firstly proposed a detailed examination of these factors. It emphasized that the government should develop measures for children who were born into poverty, or who died because of poverty. Raising funds, establishing institutions to shelter and protect poor children, and providing financial aid to families who could not afford to raise children were the other measures proposed.[42] In short, the Doctor's

Association made the following six proposals: (1) a government office should be established to impose the anti-abortion laws; (2) the abortionist should be punished; (3) the morals and manners of the children should be improved; (4) an institution to raise illegitimate Muslim children and foundlings should be established; (5) philanthropic funds should be established to protect poor children; (6) financial aid should be provided for families with more than seven children.[43]

The Ottoman government's reaction to the framework proposed by the Doctor's Association was quite positive. Throughout the rest of the nineteenth century, especially the Meclis-i Vala, the upper legislative court, showed its perspective change by initiating concrete measures. At the same time, the Ministry of the Interior formulated measures to stop abortion on more concrete grounds. During this period we see an example of increasing financial assistance for families having several children or those having twins or triplets, which was a process started much earlier.[44] In accordance with the proposal of the Doctor's Association, wages were offered to those who took care of foundlings.[45] Moreover, the exact financial source to cover this support was for the first time defined. Having a doctor's report also became obligatory for the burial of babies.[46] Finally, the opening of a poorhouse (Darülaceze) in 1896, that later started to shelter foundlings, and the Imperial Orphanage (Darülhayr-ı Ali) in 1902, to shelter orphans and foundlings can also be contextualized as part of this approach.[47]

Abortion as a Matter of Public Health

As pronatalists expressed their anxieties concerning depopulation on more concrete grounds, more developed solutions were also formulated. One of the outcomes of this shift was the inscription of abortion within the context of forensic medicine in 1871. Although the ambiguity of the term *ıskat-ı cenin* in Ottoman Turkish had not been solved, anti-abortionist doctors started to handle both abortion and miscarriage as criminal events within the purview of forensic medicine. In 1871, the Doctor's Association prepared a manual to instruct doctors on the principles of investigation and inspection in cases of wounding, murder and abortion/miscarriage. This suggests that the approach towards abortion was stripped of its moral and religious baggage and the problem was situated within everyday criminal events.[48] Furthermore, in this period, as in the case of the increased reporting of malpractice of midwives and doctors, the documentation on abortion/miscarriage became more medical and in the few cases investigated it is possible to find forensic reports attached.

An interesting example of this change is the case of Gülsüm Hanım, who voluntarily wanted the examination of the discharge she had when she was three months into her pregnancy. Most fascinatingly, Gülsüm had collected the substance she discharged in a glass jar and send it to the local police station for its examination. The police station then sent the jar to the School of Medicine and asked them to examine whether the substance in the jar really belonged to an embryo or not. They also asked whether the embryo could still maintain its vitality even if it had lost some of its part. The School of Medicine separated the substance into two, and upon analysis, it concluded that the substance was not an embryo but merely blood, and did not contain foetal tissues.[49] Although it is difficult to know the intensions of Gülsüm, she might have wanted to make sure that she did not lose her baby or to remove suspicion before somebody else raised the issue and questioned whether she had had an abortion or not.

In this period, besides being redefined within the context of forensic medicine, abortion was increasingly associated with public health. One outstanding indication of this attitude is the decree Abdülhamid II sent to the Ministry of the Interior to order the inspection of the reasons of abortion and to search for possible remedies. Upon receiving the decree, the ministry established a commission, which shortly prepared a report and sent it to the Ottoman sultan in 1890.[50] Although this report partially reiterates the perspective of the Doctor's Association, it is important for demonstrating the reception of non-official views by the government offices. The report prepared by the Ministry of the Interior also concurs that the legal sanctions of the 1858 criminal code practically remained ineffective and the abortionist was most of the time left unpunished. The commission first of all suggested the re-evaluation of the law codes. It also proposed nominating the administrative and juridical staff responsible for imposing the law locally and if they failed to apply the law, they would be punished for malpractice and ignoring their duties. This proposal was new, since for the first time the agents of the law were defined. In addition, the ministry proposed the preparation and distribution of a manual that brought forward the religious and humanitarian responsibility of condemning abortionists.[51]

Besides imposing punishments, the policy of providing financial aid to families in difficulty was also articulated. Accordingly, the commission decided to continue supporting families who had more than four children but lacked the means to raise them, with monthly stipends.[52] Moreover, in order to raise public awareness on the issue, the publication of a pamphlet was ordered for distribution in the provinces.[53] With the aim of better presenting the issue, persuading, and receiving the consent of the local people, the Ministry of the Interior decided to publish the pamphlets that were to be distributed in the Arab provinces in Arabic.[54] The novelty of this pamphlet was the way it linked abortion with hygiene, which again demonstrates the association of abortion with public health.

In this period, the upper state offices, namely the Council of State, the Council of Ministers (Meclis-i Vükela) as well as the Ministry of the Interior, increasingly handled abortion on a concrete basis defined by economic terms, ceasing to approach it from an ethical or religious dimension. Furthermore, the ministry duly embedded abortion in the context of public health, together with concerns such as improving the hygiene of dwellings, drinks and foods. Yet the documents prepared by it appropriated a highly pragmatic language utilizing prophetic words and Quran verses, reminding readers of otherworldly punishments. In other words, despite the shift of abortion into a public health context by the 1890s, practically, the Ministry of the Interior continued to invoke religious and moral sanctions, in order to attain its goals. During the reign of Abdülhamid II especially, from 1876, Quranic verses and prophetic words were widely used, which may initially seem like a return to the earlier approach in 1838. However, upon closer examination of the policies implemented to prevent abortion, we see that Abdülhamid II approached the problem from a material point of view, and his policies made a significant contribution to the redefinition of the causes of abortion on a material basis and in relation with other public health issues.[55] In this sense, I argue, although abortion was moved into the secular sphere of public health, banning abortion retained an association with profanity in this period; when it came to communicating the harms of abortion to the ordinary people, a vocabulary invoking fears of divine punishment was used.[56] The reconceptualization of abortion in this context meant that, while the bureaucrats against abortion maintained their concerns about population increase, they simultaneously developed an awareness about the protection of the good health of the extant population. Promoting population increase, removing the reasons that led to its decline and maintaining the well-being of the extant population became different faces of the same pronatalist goals.

The problematization of some people's lifestyles and the levels of healthiness in different sections of Ottoman society was another indication of the increasing attention the Ministry of the Interior gave to public health. The bureaucrats in the ministry argued that in towns, and especially in villages, the majority of dwellings were constructed without regard to health standards. Local people slept on bare soil without using mattresses, or even a thin piece of fabric. Moreover, the rural population consumed food and drink that were either soiled or with unknown contents.[57] For that reason, the Ministry of the Interior made a decision to establish mobile health units that would inspect Ottoman towns in turn. These units would contain five or six new graduates of the School of Medicine, preferably including a surgeon and a chemist, if possible. They would be supplied with the necessary devices and equipment to examine for germs. A handbook defining the rules related to the working conditions of these units would be written too. This handbook would also cover a list of sicknesses and disorders found in each specific location, as well as the possible means of their treatment.[58]

The commission formed in 1892, under the Ministry of the Interior, upon Abdülhamid's order, shortly produced a very detailed report, a declaration and a manual following the proposals and perspectives of the Ministry of Interior and the Board of Ministers.[59] The report handled abortion and hygiene as connected, as part of the same problem: the menace of the depopulation in the Ottoman Empire. The manual reiterated the offer to establish mobile health units that would examine unhygienic conditions causing the decline of the population in Ottoman towns and cities.[60] Although it did not make novel suggestions, this report, with its scope and details, demonstrates the institutionalization of the approaches towards abortion and its consolidation within the context of public health.

The report emphasized the importance of establishing mobile health units and suggested some topics for their exploration. It identified and listed these topics as questions that were to be addressed to municipal doctors, administrators, and local men and women. To give some examples, some of the following questions were asked: 'Were the women who had numerous pregnancies the majority previously?', 'Are they the majority now?', 'If such women are decreasing in number do you think that the termination of pregnancies plays a role in this change?', 'What kinds of methods and means are used to abort a foetus?', 'Which herbs or medicaments are used?', 'Are these medicines sold in the pharmacies?', and 'Are there any doctors or midwives known to help with abortions?' Besides questions about the experiences of reproduction, the doctors were supposed to query the general standards of public health in the places they were investigating. For this purpose, some of the questions asked included: 'Are the houses built in damp and dark trenches?', 'Do the houses have windows to allow air circulation?', 'Where do the local people sleep, on a mattress, a tapestry, animal fur, or on the bare soil?', 'Do they protect themselves from the sun?', 'What do they eat?', 'Do they eat an adequate amount of meat and wheat every day?', 'Do they avoid eating mildewed bread?', 'Is the nearby area swampy?', 'Is the drinking water clean?', 'What are the common diseases? Are there any common seasonal sicknesses or genetic diseases?', and 'Is syphilis common? Is small pox common?'[61]

According to the report, upon inspecting these health issues, if the health unit concluded that the population had been decreasing and that abortion was one of the reasons, it would search for the means and drugs used for it. The report also ordered the members of the mobile health unit to tell the local people, in the proper language, that exterminating a foetus was no different than homicide, even suicide since they could very possibly die trying to induce an abortion. The health unit was also supposed to write a final report presenting the reasons for the scarcity of the population and the possible remedies for it. If the health unit discovered that midwives, or other medical experts, assisted in abortions, they would be punished according to the law, regardless of their having licenses and they would be banished from practice. If the means the women used to have an abortion were sold in pharmacies, their sale would be controlled and banned. However, if the women used herbs that they picked at the countryside, the health units would find, inspect and classify those herbs. The antidotes of those herbs would also be found, according to the report.[62]

In sum, the report defined the perspectives for the search of the medical reasons for population decline. Significantly, it assumed that it was not merely abortion, but that unhealthy food, drink and housing, contagious diseases, lack of proper treatment, inattentiveness towards smallpox injections, ignorance of having a good daily rest, syphilis and the lack of its proper treatment, and failure to have a regular doctor's check- up, were all major medical reasons that led to population decline.[63] This approach explicitly indicated that abortion was a major cause, but not the single reason for the decrease in population, and the desired population increase could not be achieved by merely eliminating abortion, but should be supported by enhancing the overall measures and standards of health and sanity. It was, moreover, acknowledged that maintaining the well-being of the extant population was another big target and failing that would severely limit the success of pronatalist policies.

Is Abortion a Social or a Personal Issue?

By the end of the century, abortion became one of the most prominent hallmarks of the control of female sexuality and body. However, this control was not without limitations and contentions. Although the elite discourses were more or less consistent and comprehensive, there were also low but alternative voices raised by the ordinary people who were seen as the subjects of medical and legal bans on abortion. As discussed above, the intimate nature of the issue does not lend itself to generalizations on women's experiences of abortion. Yet, the ubiquity of documents produced by the bureaucratic and medical elites is one of the strongest evidence of the failure to discourage and limit the practice of abortion. Popular literature, despite its production by the elite writers, offers us tiny clues about the success of the anti-abortion policies and the dissenting approaches.

One of the rare examples of the popular discourses on the harms of abortion is the theatre play titled *Iskat-ı Cenin: Facia* (Abortion: A Tragedy) written by Hasan Bedrettin.[64] The play does not limit its attention to the harms of abortion but centres around several major contemporary social problems, including forced marriage and squander. Both of these topics have been major sources of controversy and it is possible to find the imprint of those social phenomena through the pages of many contemporary journals, newspapers and novels. This play demonstrates that the Ottoman elites tapped popular genres to support their legal and political combat against abortion. Moreover, it is a vivid example of the importance Ottoman intellectuals attach to popular genres and print culture to express the political and cultural contentions and to influence the society towards their solutions.

One of the protagonists of this theatre play is Afife Hanım, a young and inexperienced girl, who is expected to marry her cousin Şevki Bey whom she does not like since she in love with another young man, Hilmi Bey. Şevki is not in love with Afife either. He is a squanderer without a proper work or proper manners. As such, he is a stereotypical antagonist figure of Ottoman literature. He consumed his large inheritance recklessly and now tries to recover this loss by speculating in the newly establishing stock market. But with his financial knowledge poor, capital not so large and temperament deceivable, he shortly falls trap to bankers who lend him money with high interest rates. The only chance left to him is to marry his cousin and to own the wealth of his uncle. Indeed, most of the arranged marriages depicted by the Ottoman novelists were based on the concerns about protecting family fortunes and property. As a result, most of them resulted with unhappiness and sometimes the ruin of the couples. There are a good many number of plays and novellas criticizing forced marriage and advocating companionate marriage. It is telling in this sense that abortion and forced marriage are touched upon in the same play as two different but related social ills.

In the play, thanks to some lucky coincidences and to some tricks, Afife and Hilmi manage to marry. However, they could not escape the vengeance of Şevki when Afife becomes pregnant. The emergence of a new inheritor leads Şevki to bribe Afife's doctor and midwife to convince her to terminate her pregnancy, and Afife's wet nurse and husband are also easily manipulated by these professionals. Unable to resist them all, Afife desperately gives in to the operation induced by the midwife. However, the operation proves fatal and she pays her wrong decision with her life.

Although abortion and the tragedy it causes give its name to the play, it constitutes only the last part of the play. However, protagonists' argumentation and apprehension of abortion and the ways they justify its practice offer us unique opportunity to understand and to reconstruct contemporary approaches to abortion in Ottoman society. Different protagonists of the play have different views and hence represent different understandings. What happens at the end of the play gives clues about playwright's evaluation and judgement of those different perceptions. Afife, who is the victim of abortion, is the only person that rejects abortion without hesitation. However, she is not strong enough to conduct her own will and surrenders to his husband, and pays this with her life. Hilmi is the ambivalent character and his indecisiveness and self-persuasion represents how some people in Ottoman society decided to induce this act. Hilmi, on the one hand, believes that abortion is homicide and that it is wrong to end his child's life, which he denotes as the fruit of his own life (*semere-i hayat*). But on the other hand, he is very worried that Afife will not be able to give birth and will lose her life during parturition if not before. Although he is not comfortable with the idea, he vindicates it through the risks pregnancy and childbirth pose to his wife. After a long hesitation and ambivalence, he reaches to the conclusion that Afife's health and wellness are most important, and once she recovers they can have another baby. His argumentation about and justification of abortion reflect a widely-shared position in Ottoman society.

The pragmatic standpoint of Ottoman women is best represented by Afife's wet nurse (*kethuda*). While she is worried about Afife's health and wellness like Hilmi, she believes without any hesitation that in case one's health is at stake, there is nothing wrong with having an abortion. Although this approach was condemned by Ottoman intellectuals, it constitutes the gist of the Hanafi School of Islam's handling of abortion. As I have discussed above, abortion was not recommended or encouraged by the Hanafi law, nevertheless, it was not seen as a sin if the mother's life was at risk. Both Hilmi and Afife's wet nurse legitimize the termination of the pregnancy on the grounds of the risk it poses to the mother's health. Hasan Bedrettin, the playwright, is harsher on them compared to the bribed doctor and midwife, killing one and devastating the other at the end. The bribed doctor and midwife are the corrupted characters in the play: they are aware, deep down, that Afife's constitution is not strong enough to survive the abortion and know the vice of abortion. However, in their case, the pleasures of money offered to them in this life beat the fear of punishments in the afterlife.

The midwife in the play also reiterates some other contemporary ideas about abortion. In order to convince and comfort Afife, she tells her that many women do actually want to terminate their pregnancies to avoid the difficulties during childbirth and also the vicissitudes of childcare especially in the first few years of life. According to her, most women lose their youth and beauty after childbirth and hence the love and admiration of their husbands.[65] These ideas also represent the ways many Ottoman intellectuals evaluate the resort to abortion. As I discussed above, the practice of abortion was seen through the dichotomy of 'debauchery' (*safahat*) and 'misery' (*sefalet*) by the mainstream of Ottoman elites. This play shares this approach and criticizes women who terminate their pregnancies in order to avoid the difficulties of childcare. In a way, the corrupted midwife offers and advocates the point of view of corrupted women.

The standpoint of the midwife contrasts strongly with that of Hilmi and Afife's wet nurse. Although they sincerely care for Afife, their conclusions are wrong, and as such their role is also to show that the idea offered by religion was wrong also. In the end, despite the unfocused plot, the play concludes that there is no excuse for having an abortion and its consequence is never beneficial. According to the playwright Hasan Bedrettin, the argument 'I/we can have a child the next time' cannot be vindicated since there may never be a next time. Along these lines, this theatre play highlights the contrast between the Islamic law and Tanzimat laws concerning abortion. As such, it also challenges popular attitudes towards abortion as justified by Islamic law. Nobody in the play other than Afife worries that terminating the pregnancy is a grave sin.

Indeed, Islamic attitudes towards abortion were more liberal than the Tanzimat attitudes. While, the Hanafi school of Islam that constituted the backbone of the Ottoman legal system allowed abortion when the mother's life was at risk, the Tanzimat ideals and the secular laws banned it unconditionally. In the play as well, although Afife has some socially acceptable justifications to terminate her pregnancy, this decision did not produce propitious outcomes. If pregnancy and childbirth are risky, abortion is fatal. It never is a solution, but is the source of harm and tragedy. Maybe that is the reason why Hasan Bedreddin kills Hilmi by making him commit a suicide besides the poor Afife. The play concludes with Afife's father's devastation for losing his daughter as well as the whole family line that goes back over two centuries. Abortion leads not only the loss of life of the expectant mother and the destruction of the family, but it exterminates the whole family lineage. Thus, Hasan Bedrettin seems to imply that if Ottoman women do not stop this evil practice it will eventually lead to the extermination of the whole Turkish/Muslim population throughout the Ottoman lands. Hence according to him, abortion not only harms the people directly involved, but has even more dreadful consequences for society as a whole.

The Ottoman intellectuals were worried about the social consequences of abortion more than its personal ones. Discourses on the harm of abortion oscillate between personal and social harms of abortion, yet in the end it is always the negative impacts on the well-being of Ottoman society that makes it imperative to eradicate. In other words, although the discourses on abortion emphasized the risks of abortion on the mother's life, banning abortion was a political rather than a humanitarian goal for Ottoman intellectuals. For example, one article published in *Akile*, a women's journal published in Salonika, gives overt clues about the social ills of abortion practice.[66] This article mentions that Ottoman women terminate their pregnancies for many different reasons. In some cases, it is the husband who forces the wife to terminate her pregnancy. The burdens and difficulties of raising children and the ignorance concerning the ills of abortion are also major factors.[67] This article also talks about the different methods used to forcefully terminate pregnancies, including execution of an operation and use of chemical medicaments. Nonetheless, it warns readers that the mother will most likely lose her life and hence argues that abortion should be avoided.

A substantial part of this article is devoted to the personal and social consequences and vicissitudes of abortion. First of all, according to its writer, it is obvious that a woman who does not have pity for an innocent and beloved one, and buries her/him in the black soil before she/he could see the sun, would have no pity for her husband either. Thus, neither husbands nor other relatives could trust such pitiless women. If there is no other reason forced upon her, husbands and relatives should abandon such women when they have the opportunity.[68] However, in addition to personal ills, the articles reminds readers that abortion harms society in numerous ways. Undertaking a hypothetical argument, the article supposes that if a child were given the opportunity to live, he would grow up and contribute to his society. Killing him before he is able to grow into a full person would also stripe the society from the possible contributions he would be able to make in the future according to this hypothesis.[69]

Despite their loudness and ubiquity, the discursive and legal measures against abortion seem to remain meagre in terms of discouraging abortion and encouraging reproduction, which can also be seen from the article in *Akile*. In agreement with the archival evidence, this article also laments that the sanctions defined in the criminal code do not deter women from the crime of abortion. The limitations of contemporary legal measures drove Ottoman intellectuals to emphasize and remind women of the punishments awaiting them in the afterlife. As discussed above, a moralistic discourse emphasizing sins and eternal punishment has always been used pragmatically by Ottoman intellectuals to discourage the practice of abortion, and this approach is emphasized in this piece with a construction of an imagined scene of interrogation in the afterlife. Here the woman has no answer to justify her crime. As such she is portrayed as being no different than the 'bloody' murderers with whom she would share the same destiny.

Creating imaginary scenes with the aim of delineating the personal harms of abortion and scaring women was a common strategy shared by Ottoman writers. While the imaginary scene in *Akile* depicts an interrogation scene in the afterlife, another piece by Ahmet Rasim constructs a scene in this life.[70] Rasim's account is significant for not limiting the abortion practice to the debauchery/misery dichotomy, and for questioning whether there is a female nature or anything essential about femininity. This account starts with a description of quite an early morning. The wilderness and harshness of the nature is torn down by a woman's scream. The writer asks the readers to carefully listen to the scream. This is the scream of a woman who is trying to abort her baby. This woman, contemplates Ahmet Rasim, is aborting the baby that she has been feeding deep inside her uterus for the last two months. But she is not feeling well, her eyelashes close under the strength of the medicine, her weak nerves totally collapse as if she is on the verge of nervous breakdown. She suffers a lot. Ahmet Rasim searches for the reasons why she is so scared and paralysed. He imagines that as a purplish substance drops into the bowl in front of her, she is petrified and then her eyes are fixed into that substance so firmly that she cannot escape. Ahmet Rasim writes that although she is not fully aware, she thinks about the stolen future awaiting the deceased. If only she had given birth to him rather than aborting, she would have heard his giggles six months later, watch his childish tantrums a year later, observe his first steps, his growth, his plays and when he reaches the age of twenty she would have seen his contributions to humanity.[71]

In this piece, Ahmet Rasim concludes that a mother who imagines, for a second, the future awaiting her child, would not be able to commit such a murderous act. He believes that it is only women who are incapable of evaluating the consequences of this terrible practice, the rights of the father over the child and the harm such a murder causes humanity, who are able to commit this crime.[72]

It is also very significant that Ahmet Rasim problematizes the religious point of view. Rather than religion, he emphasizes discipline (*terbiye-i medeniye*) as the main factor to eradicate the practice of abortion from the Ottoman society. According to him, discipline is more important than religion since it is the real bond that holds society together. Civilization and discipline are used in very close meanings in this piece, and civilizing and disciplining the members of the society is seen as a humanitarian law and duty. In this framework, an important role is assigned to the mothers, who are supposed to watch and inspect closely those members of the society who may be prone to practise abortion. It is the mothers' duty to protect the society from the harms of abortion. The emphasis made on discipline ties the issue of abortion to the politics of female body. As I will discuss in the following chapter, an important register of Ottoman pronatalism and politics of female body was the emergence of medical discourses on pregnancy. Those discourses which become most overt in prescriptive books for pregnant women were indeed narratives of discipline. According to Ottoman intellectuals, this discipline seems to be the medicament for the habit of terminating pregnancies, too.

Besides the female nature, Ahmet Rasim also questions marriage and the norms concerning intimacy. He argues that if a policeman happens to gaze secretly into the houses, he would see that houses are scenes of numerous crimes. It is in the closeness of this private space that many crimes and murderous acts are committed. According to him, marriage is no longer serving its purpose: the reproduction of children.

The debate about abortion also brings questions about the female nature and femininity. While Ahmet Rasim makes some essentialist generalizations about female nature, he concludes with negative and controversial conclusions. Counter-arguing the widespread association of affection and tenderness with women, he reminds readers that it is in fact women who murder their children before they are born.[73] It is not only Ahmet Rasim who makes essentialist judgements about female nature; a very prominent Ottoman intellectual, Namık Kemal, also shares a similar point of view. Namık Kemal wrote several articles on population and was one of the most ardent opponents of abortion.[74] He was not only critical about women who avoid having children due to debauchery; he also disapproved of women who practise abortion due to poverty.[75] Namık Kemal first criticizes that the very same women who cry for many years for a baby they lost after three days of life do not hesitate or feel any guilt when it comes to abortion. Maybe the most stringent opposition to the practice of abortion is raised with his question, 'Why does a mother, who does not hesitate to kill the innocent in her womb, avoid eating her children just like a cat after they were born?' Indeed, Namık Kemal uses very harsh vocabulary to describe the experiences of women who terminate their pregnancies. He compares these women with snakes and scorpions and concludes that they are worse than such creatures. Moreover, he claims that such women cannot be believers since they do not fear God or the prophet. And he does not only target his harsh criticisms at women, but some men receive their share too. For example, Namık Kemal mentions that in Ottoman society there are also men who impregnate their female slaves (*cariye*) and then who kill both slave and child.

Yet Namık Kemal's argument clearly emphasizes female debauchery as the main reason behind abortion. He criticizes women for poisoning their children with opium so that they will not wake up throughout the night. Such women undergo abortions just to avoid the burden of carrying the foetus in their womb for a few months. Finally, he again compares mothers having abortions with wild beasts, and says that although the wildest animal, the lion, does not commit this crime, human mothers, associated with affection, do, attacking their beloved unborn children against the wish of God.

Abortion and Demographic Prospects

So far this chapter has presented the anti-abortion debate within the context of nineteenth-century anxieties regarding population decline. However, the very important question concerning the definition of population has, for the most part, remained untouched. When they were articulating their concerns about the fate of the population and combating depopulation, the bureaucrats and medical elites who were opposing abortion were not actually worried about maintaining the extant demographic composition, but their attention was limited to Muslim groups within the empire. As a result, starting from the early 1860s, the process to engender Ottomans was formulated by them on more refined grounds, broadening the populationist goals from merely the numerical quantity to the definition of who an 'Ottoman' was. Although this definition was not strictly and decisively made, I submit that being an Ottoman was increasingly associated with being Muslim.

One of the earlier indications of this attitude can be found in one of the contemporary positivist journals, *Mecmua-i Fünun* (Journal of Sciences) that sporadically devoted its pages to medicine.[76] In its December 1866 issue the doctor Kırımlızade Aziz İdris Bey wrote a piece on abortion and the harm it causes.[77] Doctor Aziz was a military physician who specialized in pathology and internal medicine. He played an important role in the struggle to make Turkish rather than French the official language of instruction of medicine. As such he took part in the establishment of the Imperial Faculty of Medicine (Mekteb-i Tıbbiye-i Mülkiye) and became its first director.[78] He was also one of the defenders of contemporary pronatalist views. In his article, he reasserted that the grandeur and glory of a country depended on the abundance of its population. According to Doctor Aziz, contributing to population increase was the duty and responsibility of every individual. Expending efforts to this purpose would bring even more prosperity and power than conquering other countries. Aziz gave a prominent place to abortion in accordance with nineteenth-century assumptions.[79] He also reported in detail about the harms and methods of abortion.[80]

In this article, Aziz explicitly demonstrated that he was specifically worried about the fate of the Muslim population rather than the extant demographic composition of the Ottoman society. According to the doctor, since it was Muslim women who frequently practised abortion, it was the Muslim population that declined. And he lamented that since non-Muslim women did not practise abortion, the populations of non-Muslims communities were not decreasing but, on the contrary, were increasing. To underline his concerns about the depopulation risk for Muslims, Aziz also remonstrated that military duty was only performed by the Muslim population, and hence led to further loss of Muslim lives during the times of war. In this sense, Aziz's framework was shaped by the assumption that the Muslim population was declining due to abortion and military duty, whereas the Christian population enjoyed growth by being devoid of these two factors.[81]

In order to demonstrate the huge costs of abortion on the prospects of the Muslim population, Aziz made some calculations. Assuming that the fecundity age for women was between fifteen and forty-five, in Istanbul, and assuming there were approximately 150,000 Muslim women between these ages, he calculated that 150,000 pregnancies would be terminated in thirty years if each and every woman dropped one baby throughout her overall fertile period. Assuming that only one Muslim person died in Istanbul a day, he calculated that approximately 400 people would die in a year, and 144,000 in thirty years. Aziz compared both estimations and concluded that the loss of lives due to abortion in one year was much higher than the lives lost with normal deaths. Of course, not only were his assumptions completely arbitrary, but his calculations were also wrong. Yet, Aziz's mindset and argument opened the passageway for the growing interest in the definition of the population. His persistent emphasis on 'Muslim' women suggests that he was not worried about the fate of the overall population, but merely that of Muslims.[82]

The Ministry of the Interior also shared this attitude as evinced by an 1890 decree about abortion. In an unusual way, the decree produced by the ministry started with reference to a letter that was alleged to have been sent by someone who had travelled around İzmid, Bursa, and the villages around Istanbul with his wife. According to the anonymous writer of the letter, in the villages they had visited they observed that women who had two or at most three children tried to have abortions when they conceived once again. In order to abort their children, they boiled the stems of some herbs, drank it and very easily terminated their pregnancies. The writers relates how his wife had for some time mixed among such women and observed how the locals procured such herbs, prepared abortifacient drugs and dropped their babies. According to their observations, four in every twenty women who tried to have an abortion died, since in Karamürsel, in one year's time, twenty abortions took place and four of them resulted in the death of the mother. To add more sorrow, those practising abortion were solely Muslim women, and one of the primary reasons pushing them to terminate their pregnancies was their poverty. Unfortunately, the Muslim population steadily decreased due to conscription on the one hand, and women avoiding giving birth on the other, whereas Christian villages developed and prospered because of the lack of these two unfavourable factors.[83]

Finally, it is possible to trace the anxieties about the widespread practice of abortion among Muslim women of the empire in contemporary popular narratives.[84] In addition to the legal grounds, the struggle to ban abortion was carried out on popular grounds. While the Ottoman ruling power searched for ways to discourage women to practise abortion by outlawing it and by offering policies to encourage them to give birth, it also received the direct and indirect help of Ottoman intellectuals who argued against abortion in popular literature.[85] However, popular literature gives us significant clues about the presuppositions and ideological premises of the Ottoman intellectuals. For example, both the theatre play *Iskat-ı Cenin. Facia* (Abortion. A Tragedy),[86] which lamented the social and personal ills brought about by abortion and has been published and recited in the late 1870s, and the novel *Sefile* (The Wretched Girl)[87] published in 1885, depicted how young girls were ruined as the result of abortion. It is not mere coincidence that the protagonists of both works are Muslim girls. Similar to the official and elite discourses, the popular genres and narratives also underlined anxieties concerning the practices of abortion among Muslim women.

When the anxieties about the fate of the Muslim population is contextualized within the population movements and demographic transformations in this period, it is striking to see that the Muslim population actually experienced a slightly increased birth rate in the second half of the nineteenth century,[88] and its overall share in the total demographic composition increased significantly due to the migration of Muslim populations after the Crimean War, and the sharp drop of the Christian population mainly due to the loss of territories. The incompatibility between what was actually taking place and what was proposed in official and non-official documents should, thus, be considered from the political standpoints and agendas of Ottoman pronatalists. In this sense, the pronatalism of the nineteenth century, and the battle to increase the Ottoman population, was in fact about engendering a Muslim population. Even though the Muslim population did not seem to be threatened in the first place, the demographic turbulence of the nineteenth century led Ottoman government officials to become worried about its fate. In other words, the fear of the decline of the Muslim population cannot be understood on a concrete quantitative basis, but becomes meaningful in the ideological context of the nineteenth century. Despite the promises of the Tanzimat Rescript for the equality of Muslims and non-Muslims alike, the social hierarchies formed over centuries hindered the construction of a common cultural identity. The Tanzimat Rescript promised equality of all Ottoman subjects before the law, regardless of their faith, and the protection of their life, property and dignity. However, the loss of the predominantly non-Muslim territories, on the one hand, and the migration of Muslims, on the other, significantly restructured the demographic composition on behalf of the Muslim population. This demographic transformation seriously abridged the Tanzimat ideals by eroding their material base. The Ottoman pronatalists referred solely to the Muslim population when they were worried about demographic prospects. I argue that they were solely anxious that it was the 'Muslim' population that was decreasing, and lamented that the non-Muslim and especially Christian populations were on the increase.

The examination of abortion legislation and the attitudes towards abortion mirrors the ways the Ottoman state approached its population as well as female sexuality. Although initially the government offices discussed abortion solely through a moralistic and religious perspective, they eventually changed their outlook and searched for the reasons that led women to terminate unwanted pregnancies, and accordingly, sought remedies to discourage them. The elaboration of the anti-abortion debate, and the search for the legal, medical and discursive means to prevent abortion, illustrate the politicization of sexuality in this period. In this chapter, I have showed that the choice to give or not to give birth was a political issue in the mid- to late nineteenth-century Ottoman society. As such, I have offered an alternative account of the transformations during the nineteenth century, one that re-evaluates the renowned stories from the perspective of gender. While the Ottoman state tried to medicalize childbirth and pregnancy, it also tried to discourage Ottoman women from having abortions. In addition to raising the standards during, before and after childbirth, it tried to diminish the need to have abortions by offering monetary incentives. Although state encroachment upon the sphere of female sexuality is indisputably oppressive in many respects, within the specificities of the nineteenth century, it also demonstrates the ways the Ottoman state was giving increasing attention to its female subjects. It was in this period that Ottoman women first became legal agents and were addressed directly by the state. In this sense, I suggest that this process could not be stigmatized as absolute control over female bodies, but entailed opportunities for women's agency. To make it more specific, in return for bearing the children needed for a prosperous country, women received their share in the promised redefinition of the relationship between the Ottoman state and society.

4 PREGNANCY AS A SITE OF MEDICAL INTERVENTION

This chapter investigates the medicalization and reconceptualization of pregnancy towards the end of the nineteenth century. In the previous two chapters, I examined the attempts to promote increased birth rates and to decrease maternal and infant death rates within the broader framework of Ottoman pronatalism. In order to achieve these goals, and in order to provide enhanced health services to Ottoman women during childbirth, the Ottoman state first sought to establish a medical basis through educating and licensing midwives and structuring a medical hierarchy. Simultaneously, as part of the combat against population decline, abortion was banned on the premises that it was the main factor responsible for the diminishing Ottoman population. Once these initial policies had been implemented, Ottoman pronatalists turned their attention to women, and initiated policies to regulate their maternal capability.

In this chapter I will shift my concentration away from the institutional and legal fields focused on in the Chapter 2 and 3, and turn to the rest of society, in order to analyse the medical and discursive ground on which the pronatalist battle was fought. This chapter discusses the subjection of pregnancy and childbirth to medical scrutiny. Despite the discourses emphasizing the benevolence, mercy and affection of the Ottoman sultan, decreasing the maternal and infant death rates, and saving the mothers' and children's lives, was not merely a humanitarian, but a political issue, in the Ottoman Empire. As I have elaborated on above, there was a broad consensus between state authorities and Ottoman medical elites that population was a crucial component of the economic wealth and political power of the country. The policies directed towards the medicalization of childbirth, professionalization of midwifery and the bans on abortion were formulated within this context. However, one major linchpin of Ottoman pronatalism was the control of female sexuality and the female body. Hence, it is vital for this work to analyse the discourses and policies related to disciplining the female body, which was defined by the protonalist intellectuals mostly by its maternal function and ability to reproduce. According to them, the female body was meant for reproduction and for producing offspring. Thus, it should be disciplined with these functions in mind. This discipline obviously became utmost important during pregnancy. According to this view, pregnancy should be controlled – or at least monitored – by medical experts, and childbirth should take place in a medicalized environment. Especially towards the end of the century, voices were more vociferously raised to draw attention to the need for maternity hospitals that would provide practical training alongside theoretical instruction, especially for medical students.

Along with the attempts to open maternity hospitals, the medicalization of childbirth was sought on discursive grounds. It is in this period that the first examples of prescriptive books for expectant mothers were published. Besides giving admonitions to expecting mothers during their pregnancy, these books offered a prolific ground to express and diffuse pronatalist ideals. They were not only about the right health care during pregnancy, but the normative literature contributed to reconstructing the female experience of pregnancy. An examination of the prescriptive literature targeting pregnant women helps us to understand the premises and complexities of Ottoman pronatalism especially when taken together with the regulation of midwifery, broader medical developments in obstetrics and anti-abortion campaigns. Moreover, an investigation into the prescriptive literature demonstrates the mutuality of the medical, legal and institutional transformations with the discursive changes, and hence makes overt the new role given to Ottoman women as the producers of population. These prescriptive manuals were not only about health care during pregnancy; they were closely intertwined with the transformation of midwifery practices, and the legal and medical attempts to control female sexuality. While medical and institutional developments changed the practices of childbirth, the appearance of written work on pregnancy, parturition and ante-natal care contributed to the reconceptualization of the female experiences wrapped around childbirth. As the century reached a close, the changes in childbirth practices and the emergence of new discourses, when taken together, point to a reconceptualization of the female body. That new female body was predominantly defined by its ability to give birth and to rear children.

The examination of the prescriptive literature on pregnancy offers us valuable insights to reconstruct the feminine bodily experience, which we will never recover completely. Yet the importance of its analysis becomes overt, especially when we consider the lack of documents produced by women describing how they felt or experienced their bodies. While the prescriptive literature has limitations due to its normative content, it is still very helpful in unfolding and discussing gender relations.

As I mentioned previously, the scholarship on the history of childbirth and pregnancy in the Ottoman context awaits further development. However, as opposed to the lacuna of serious scholarly work in the field of history, popular ethnographic histories related to the customs of pregnancy and childbirth have been more warmly welcomed.[1] More serious scholarly ethnographic work has also devoted chapters to childbirth related topics. For example, an ethnographic work about Armenian village life in the eastern parts of Anatolia before 1914, devotes a full chapter to a depiction of the customs, practices and ceremonies related to pregnancy and childbirth.[2] This work, which is based on interviews with Armenian immigrants living in Detroit at the time of the research, provides rich evidence about the social practices related to pregnancy, childbirth and childcare among Armenian women of the Ottoman Empire. Carol Delaney's seminal ethnographic study, *The Seed and the Soil* (1991) also discusses the symbolic meanings of birth in Anatolian culture.[3] Delaney argues that in order to understand the mechanisms of subordination of women in monotheistic societies, one has to examine the processes and cultures of procreation. She elaborately discusses the social practices related to childbirth, the practices of midwifery, the medical and social roles of the midwives, and the ceremonies following childbirth in the specific context of a central Anatolian village. This research provides rich ethnographic data, and despite its focus on contemporary Anatolia, it is thought-provoking for historical research.

The scholarship on women's history and gender theory has produced a substantial literature to guide research on the history of pregnancy and childbirth. After the 1980s, as women and gender historians came to discuss the social control of birth and reproduction, they also handled the social history of pregnancy as a legitimate topic of historical research. The early scholarship tended mostly to idealize past times, arguing that pregnancy was treated as a 'natural' process and was controlled only by women. However, much recent scholarship has drawn attention to the limitations of such a framework and highlighted the complexities of the experience and the management of pregnancy for women of the early modern society.[4] It reconstructed the ways women of the earlier centuries discussed and shared their own experiences and understandings of pregnancy and childbirth.[5] This approach has challenged the idea that childbirth was an exclusively female culture by demonstrating that husbands also played participatory roles during pregnancy and childbirth through sharing their wives' understanding of their bodily needs, and nurturing, entertaining and comforting them. Rather than focusing solely on discourses about the physical weaknesses of women, women's and gender historians reconstructed the strategies through which women enjoyed pregnancy as a source of female strength.[6] Using hitherto untapped sources, including tracts on gynaecology and obstetrics, they deepened our understanding of the specificity of the maternal experience.[7] Women and gender historians, moreover, subsumed the ways in which medical doctors and midwives expressed their views about pregnancy and female nature in gendered ways.[8] They demonstrated that as male physicians portrayed the pregnant body in medical ways, they handled pregnancy as a project requiring proper discipline, not only from external medical forces, but also from pregnant women.[9] Along these lines, gender historians examined the prescriptive literature on pregnancy and childbirth to demonstrate the complexities of the discourses and their contribution to the redefinition of the female body.[10] They showed that the prescriptive literature, and the new discourses on pregnancy and female body, were both empowering and oppressive at the same time, and while it placed stringent demands on women, through controlling and disciplining their bodies and emotions, the advice literature also attributed agency and responsibility to pregnant bodies.[11]

In light of the scholarship on women's and gender history I scrutinize how pregnancy guidebooks functioned to *order* or *govern* female bodies, and I elaborate on the ways in which these prescriptive books structured femininity. However, I also point out the opportunities they created for women's agency. Although it is true that these documents constructed female bodies as mediums to be regulated, disciplined and shaped, it is again through such documents that women of the nineteenth century gained historical agency. The maternal body of the expectant mother was not merely a site of state intervention, but the mother was also primarily responsible for raising healthy children. While the female body became increasingly defined by its reproductive capacities, it was, in the last analysis, the women themselves who were to govern their bodies.

Pregnancy Manuals and the Maternal Body

While the Ottoman medical experts were trying to establish institutions that would, in the long run, medicalize childbirth, they were also medically encroaching upon the period of gestation and trying to regulate pregnancy. However, in a period when the number of male obstetricians still remained very low, the major means of advocating medical scrutiny during pregnancy was by writing about its benefits. From the 1880s on, the first examples of medical treatises concerning pregnancy and childbirth started to appear. One of the first printed books on obstetrics, *Fenn-i Vilade* (The Science of Birth), in Ottoman Turkish was published in 1880/1.[12] This book was a translation of a German physician and male-midwife, *Skanzoni*'s medical tract. The book was translated by a group of translators, İbrahim Atafi, Hüseyin Ramiz, Nafiz Serya, Hüseyin Sabri and Ahmed Hilmi. However, it was not translated directly from German, but from its edition in French. The treatise was meant to be used in obstetrics courses at the School of Medicine, and accordingly used very scholarly language that targeted medical students. One of the most outstanding aspects of this book is the absence of images and visual materials, which constitutes a contrast when compared to the treatises that appeared later in the century. As I pointed out in the previous chapters, learning obstetrics without actually conducting any births meant that the medical students at the start of their careers, had in fact fewer skills than midwives who lacked theoretical instruction but had considerable hands-on expertise. Since they could not claim supremacy over midwives on the bases of practical experience, the medical men boldly underscored their mastery of medical texts and theoretical information to justify their proficiency.

The first prescriptive book counselling the right care during gestation was published only a few years after the appearance of the first medical treatise. *Haml- ü Vaz'ı Haml* (Pregnancy and Childbirth), was a translation by Halid Ziya (Uşaklıgil), one of the most prominent intellectual figures of the late nineteenth century.[13] Halid Ziya stated in the preface that he had selected and translated the parts that related to pregnancy from the work on hygiene by Auguste Debay, a French doctor and man of science. Although he did not specify the full name of the book, the translated parts had presumably been selected from Debay's best selling *Hygiène et physiologie du mariage: Histoire naturelle et médicale de l'homme et de la femme mariés dans ses plus curieux détails* (Hygiene and Marital Physiology: Natural and Medical History of the Married Man and Woman in Its Most Curious Details).[14]

Almost a decade after this first pregnancy handbook, the second example of this genre, Besim Ömer's manual, *Gebelik ve Gebelikte Tedabir* (Pregnancy and the Precautions during Pregnancy) arrived in 1900/1.[15] *Gebelik ve Gebelikte Tedabir* was the first book in Besim Ömer's series on healthcare and hygiene before, during, and after childbirth. The second volume of this series, *Doğururken ve Doğurduktan Sonra* (During and after Childbirth), concerns safety during parturition and post-natal care, and the third book, *Sıhhatnüma-yı Nevzad* (Newborn Care), handles infant care. Although we do not have specific information about the number of copies printed and sold, the existence of later editions and the multiple numbers of reprints for each book suggest that they were widely sold and read.[16] The announcement of Besim Ömer's *Gebelik ve Gebelikte Tedabir* (Pregnancy and the Precautions during Pregnancy) with quite an appreciation in one of the elite but long lived contemporary journals, *Servet-i Fünun* (Wealth of the Sciences), is another sign of the welcoming audience pregnancy manuals received.[17] This short review article praises Besim Ömer and his book quite highly. It also includes some excerpts from Besim Ömer's book. The announcement of this prescriptive book in the journal shows the importance attached to pronatalism by the contemporary intellectuals.

Haml-ü Vaz'-ı Haml is a smaller book of eighty-one pages.[18] The parts that had been translated covered proper health care during pregnancy and major medical risks during gestation and childbirth. Some popular issues, such as the safety of sexual intercourse during gestation, craving and mood swings were also handled. In addition to pregnant women, this manual also targeted expectant fathers and sporadically referred directly to them. *Gebelik ve Gebelikte Tedabir* is a larger book with 101 regular sized pages. This book deals more elaborately with the proper lifestyle of pregnant women, devoting almost seventy pages – more than half of its total size – to the hygiene, diet, entertainment, bathing and dress of expectant mothers.

The validity of the medical information included in these books is out of the scope of this chapter, yet *Gebelik ve Gebelikte Tedabir* has a more scientific outlook than *Haml-ü Vaz'-ı Haml*, both with its contents and its approach. For example, in *Gebelik ve Gebelikte Tedabir*, Besim Ömer consistently formulated his arguments through a discussion, comparison and evaluation of the approaches of prominent medical men and philosophers such as Aristotle, Avicenna (*İbn-i Sina*) and Rhazes (*İbn-i Razi*). He rarely mentions his own experiences, and when he does, he presents them as scientific observations. *Haml-ü Vaz'-ı Haml*, on the contrary, mostly has a casual and colloquial style and only rarely refers to renowned medical men. The medical complications and risks during pregnancy and childbirth, the importance of diet, or the necessity of regular health checks are handled in a more scientific manner in Besim Ömer's guide, with reference to the reasons and consequences of certain behaviours. In *Haml-ü Vaz'-ı Haml*, however, we do not find such argumentation.

Although it is never mentioned explicitly, the examples used and the admonitions given hinted that the books' audience was upper-class urban women. Besim Ömer, for example, discusses whether it is appropriate to play the piano or ride a horse during pregnancy. These entertaining activities were clearly the privilege of upper-class women. The ornaments decorating the bedroom of the expectant mother, such as laced bedspreads, heavy curtains, massive furniture and the lace covering them, also delineate a bedroom in an affluent house. Finally, not only was literacy a privilege of upper-class women in nineteenth-century Ottoman society, but these women were presumably both more open to try new medical developments and new lifestyles recommended, and had the financial means to try them when they wanted to do so.

The pregnancy manuals of the nineteenth century counselled pregnant women on how to take care of their bodies, protect their and their babies' health during gestation, and have a safe childbirth. These books also briefly covered post-natal care. However, early mothering and infant care were usually handled in separate books. In contrast to the textbooks and medical treatises on this subject, the advice manuals employed a rather normative language that not only prescribed one single correct method to be followed during pregnancy, but also made judgements for failing to follow the advice given. As another literary strategy, these manuals persistently referred to science, natural laws, human nature, as well as humanity, virtue and religious obligation as the source of their counsel. As a result, the admonitions within them gained further legitimacy and expectant mothers were left with no choice but to follow them. From this perspective, the positivist outlook of these manuals and their belief in science are in sharp contrast with the call for obedience.

The language used in these books is normative, especially in the introductory parts of the manuals, where the discourse on the obligations of the expectant mother to order her body was structured. Moreover, the introductions of both manuals are about nothing but discipline: bodily discipline and moral discipline. The health, constitution and character of the children, they maintained, was dependent on the bodily discipline of the mother. Therefore, a mother who wanted to raise a well-behaved child should first discipline her own body, and then that of her child, starting from conception. Governing her body would not only guarantee good health for herself, but for her child too.[19]

According to Besim Ömer, the effort spent in disciplining the female body was the best effort spent in the services of civilization, the most sacred of duties for humanity and the one most deserving of attention and gratitude among the services for social and moral progress. This approach takes the family as the basic unit of society and argues that mothers are the most crucial tie holding the family together.[20] Since family means mother, according to this framework, the happiness of the family depends on the discipline of the mother.[21] The health, body and character of children depend on the health of the mother, and improving her health and governing her body would, at the same time, contribute to the well-being of her children. Taking part in the formation of the bodily and the moral discipline of a young girl was highly praised by Besim Ömer, since that girl would develop into a young woman and then a mother, her discipline would pass to her children through her motherhood. Her entire family, in particular, and the whole society, in general, would benefit from her well-founded body and spirit.[22]

According to Besim Ömer's framework, discipline of the body preceded moral discipline, since the latter could only be established after achieving the former completely and competently.[23] Without first disciplining the body, moral discipline would not be possible. In other words, only a healthy, disciplined body would retain the proper moral qualities. Of course, the body at stake was the maternal body, i.e. the body designed and meant for reproduction.

The inability to give birth was the worst of all the calamities a woman could experience. In the words of Besim Ömer, it was 'like a wound that incessantly bleeds to intoxicate and reinjure itself'. This suffering was so great; one feels it as if God had placed an empty cradle that cannot bear being empty on the lap of women.[24] It is not surprising that within this framework the choice not to give birth was completely out of question in this framework. According to Besim Ömer, only immoral women tried to escape their duty to raise children, and these women could not even be accepted as women. In the cases where they did conceive, such women tried to murder their babies by abortion. Both books established a direct connection between morality and reproduction. Moral women bore children and disciplined both their bodies and those of their children as an indication of their morality, whereas immoral women failed to do so.

In order to discipline the maternal body, precise and elaborate rules to organize daily life, diet and sleep were defined in both books. The way a pregnant woman should decorate her room, organize her daily routines, the proper entertainment that she could safely enjoy, the healthy ways to dress and to do housework were all described in detail. Even the most basic issues such as how often a pregnant woman should bathe, how many times she should rub herself, the length of bathing, the warmth and even the exact temperature of the water are scrupulously described. The idea that the expectant mother should also restructure her lifestyle and routines was the substance of these counsels.

This advice was part of the attempt to strip pregnancy of its social content and to medicalize it. Pregnancy was no longer considered to be a significant component of the female social experience; it had become a period in the female life cycle which should be checked and controlled or, at the very least, monitored by physicians. Expectant mothers should put their former routines and daily practices aside and adopt healthier ways to dress, eat and amuse themselves. Their former ways of decorating their house or having any social exchange with their friends were all scorned. It was stridently announced that old habits should be replaced with healthier ones.

Although, in these texts, the habits and routines of women were denigrated, and the discourse sought to replace them with a healthier lifestyle as prescribed by obstetricians, it is crucial not to read these texts as absolute sites of dominance over female bodies. Despite the detailed nature of such admonitions, these books in fact described the principles of a healthy lifestyle and left the decision of how to structure and achieve that lifestyle on a daily basis to expectant mothers. As such, these books assigned an important degree of agency to women who followed the advice given. Moreover, women who could reorganize their daily lives according to the recommendations of the books were seen as partners of the doctors and hence appreciated.

However, this situation made the role of the medical experts slightly ambivalent. On the one hand, the role of monitoring the expectant mother and to help her have a healthy pregnancy and a healthy child was attributed to the physician. On the other hand, women were expected to take charge of their lives and redesign their daily routines. The doctors' roles, therefore, have to be sought, not in the formation of routines, but in the cases of complications. The books mention that doctors have expertise in several issues that women could not master themselves. First of all, although the common signs of pregnancy, such as changes in the breasts, missed menstrual periods, growing abdomen, nausea, vomiting and fainting, pigmentation around the nipple and feeling the movements of the baby, could be observed by everybody, the reliable signs, such as the heartbeat of the child and movements inside the abdomen, could only be diagnosed by physicians. In addition, changes in the maternal body showed merely the presence of pregnancy, but whether the baby was healthy and living could only be tested by a doctor.[25] Secondly, since the humours of the maternal body underwent major transformations during gestation, the limbs, especially the liver and the kidneys, failed to fulfil their functions properly, and made the maternal body more vulnerable to all kinds of diseases. The doctors could diagnose and cure such problems at the right time. Moreover, it was crucial to determine the position of the baby before parturition. If the head of the baby presented itself first, then a midwife might safely assist in childbirth, but breech babies, especially those who were positioned on one side rather than on the feet or on the buttocks, could only be delivered by a physician. Only a physician would know how to manoeuvre the baby in the uterus and deliver her safely.[26]

The manuals assert that although pregnancy was not a state of illness, it was a stage in the female life cycle rife with bodily and mental risks. If not handled and managed properly, according to the manuals, these risks might cost the life of the mother and the baby. Leaving a doctor's intervention to the last minute, when the illness became grave, was a huge risk to take, and early diagnosis was vital for minimizing life threatening conditions. According to this approach, the doctor's role was broadened to cover normal and healthy pregnancies, as well, and was no longer limited to difficult births and serious complications during or after delivery.

The discourse emphasizing the risks during pregnancy and the benefits of a doctor's intervention in order to minimize them is contextualized within the medical and institutional developments that redefined the role of midwives. Parallel to the approach that predominated in the second half of the nineteenth century, Besim Ömer frequently reiterated that the midwife should avoid handling complications by herself, but should call a doctor in the case of even the slightest doubt.[27] As I discussed in Chapter 1, as one of the pioneers of male midwives, as well as the major initiator of 'modern' midwifery education in the Ottoman Empire, Besim Ömer had actively sought to denigrate the role of local midwives and glorify that of obstetricians. In his various medical work, as well as advice books for midwives, he emphasized similar ideas to redraw the boundaries of midwifery practice.

Haml-ü Vaz'ı Haml, which was not written with such concerns, but rather aimed to be a bestseller, approaches midwives in a notably different way than did *Gebelik ve Gebelikte Tedabir*. This book assigned a rather positive role to midwives and talks about them quite appreciatively. Especially in the final part of the manual, *Vaz'ı hamlin müddetleri* (The Stages of Parturition), where the mechanics of childbirth were described, midwives were seen as the primary assistants of birth. First and foremost, they were seen as being responsible in cases of possible complications. Their duties, responsibilities and services were identified. Instead of urging midwives to call doctors in case of the slightest problem, this book told them how to take charge of the childbirth and handle complications. Their function was seen as useful as that of doctors' and hence, as much respected. If the 'other' was the midwife in *Gebelik ve Gebelikte Tedabir*, it was the 'old crone' in *Haml-ü Vaz'ı Haml*. The old crone was the representative of superstition and fallacy. All their doings were against reason and wisdom and hence one should turn a deaf ear to their blabber and chatter and should resist them with dignity and precaution.[28]

This way, a dichotomous opposition between superstition and reason, between quacks and medicine, female assistance and doctor's interference was established.

Another issue where the new conception of maternity can be observed wrapped into the above dichotomous framework is in nursing. *Gebelik ve Gebelikte Tedabir* underscored that breastfeeding the baby was an obligation of human nature, humanity, virtue and religion. According to this book, a woman who did not breastfeed her baby was not a complete mother. Motherhood was not merely giving birth; it also included breastfeeding and raising a child. Failing to breastfeed the baby when the mother did not have a proper excuse recognized by a physician was intolerable. According to the manuals, breastfeeding when the mother had either some sort of illness, or insufficient milk to feed the baby was seen as selfishness that would throw the life of an innocent baby into risk.

Moreover, both books drew strong parallels between milk and blood.[29] Milk was a purified or refined form of postpartum blood. During gestation, mothers fed their babies with their blood, and after parturition with their milk. Both writers asserted that milk was a sacred food and every mother's milk was designed uniquely for her child. It contained the best of whatever the infant needed.[30] From this perspective, wet nursing was, therefore, intolerable. It was not only against humanity, but was in opposition to maternal compassion and affection. However, both books lamented that the sale of that 'perfect and delicate food' in the free market was in no way rare in Ottoman society. According to the books, no mother had the right to sell her milk and deprive her own baby. Similarly, no mother had the right to give her infant another person's milk that would never nourish it properly. However, in the end, it was the wet nurses and not the middle-class women who hired them, that were to be condemned and dishonoured. Here parallels are drawn between the 'old crone' and the wet nurse as the opponent of science and reason. Again expectant mothers are placed, at their expense, beside doctors – but only, of course on the condition that they follow instructions.

One of the few topics in which fathers came into the picture was sexual intercourse during gestation. Both manuals agree that sexual intercourse during pregnancy, especially after the sixth month might be harmful to the baby. Yet, *Gebelik ve Gebelikteki Tedabir* had an objective, whereas *Haml-ü Vaz'ı haml* had a moralistic approach. In *Haml-ü Vaz'ı haml* sexual intercourse during pregnancy was seen as a failure to control one's desires and emotions. In this way, it was considered an act of people inferior to animals. Besim Ömer, however, approached the question of sexual intercourse during pregnancy from a different perspective. According to him, sexual intercourse might lead to miscarriage in the first three months,[31] and it might hurt the uterus and lead to a miscarriage in the last trimester. He therefore concluded that having intercourse was unsafe during pregnancy.[32] To him, the first right of the child was to come into the world safely,[33] and mothers were held primarily responsible for avoiding sexual intercourse.[34]

The cost of inattentiveness to hygiene and health care during pregnancy, the failure to discipline the body – essentially, the failure to obey the advice in these manuals – was rather high. Such ignorance would lead to miscarriage, early birth or unhealthy infants. The manuals proclaimed that although every mother hoped for the beauty and health of her child, this expectation only came true through total obedience to the rules of hygiene. Following the rules of hygiene obviously meant following the advice in the manuals. The manuals warned that mothers who failed to adopt the proper lifestyles presented in these manuals would not escape giving birth to babies who, at best, suffered defects and deformities.[35] The wording of these manuals puts responsibility for stillbirths and other problems directly onto the mother very explicitly.

Conversely, the more ordered the mother, the healthier and more perfect the baby. The books argued that the duties and obligations of motherhood started with conception. Once the woman felt another life developing in her own body, she should start considering herself a mother, and devote her entire activities to the happiness, needs and health of that life.[36] And until a child was able to take responsibility for their own personal hygiene, it was the responsibility of the mother to care for it.[37]

The guidebooks emphasized that expectant mothers should devote all her efforts to the well-being of her maternal body. Only by doing so would traits, such as grace, strength and good health be secured.[38] Although every mother hoped for the beauty and physical wellness of her child, that expectation came true only through total obedience to the rules of hygiene, i.e. to the advice in this book. Mothers who failed to follow the necessary precautions and rules, those who failed to change their lifestyles according to the needs of pregnancy, risked unsafe deliveries and the health of themselves and their child.

Besides repeatedly stressing these two major risks, both manuals devoted separate sections to miscarriage and pre-term labour. According to *Haml-ü Vaz'-ı Haml*, miscarriage and pre-term labour could be caused either by strong emotions or by physical factors. As mentioned above, a pregnant woman was open to extreme emotions, which, according to the advice manuals, would destroy her and hurt the baby. The physical factors might be old age, character, personality disorders, wrong (i.e. disordered) dress, diet and lifestyle, heredity or internal diseases.[39] Those who wanted to evade the great risks of miscarriage, or pre-term labour, should strictly obey the information and advice provided; otherwise, in the words used in the manuals, mothers expecting to harvest the best product of their life would gain nothing but a lifeless corpse.[40]

Since the pregnant woman was driven by her humors, she could not easily control her feelings. Especially towards the end of the term, she began to show ambivalent feelings, oscillating between misery and euphoria. She tended to exaggerate even the slightest events and became desperate and sore for nothing. In order to help her, her husband and others should have treated her like a small child, told her charming stories, funny events and jokes, and tried to relieve and change her gloomy mood.[41] *Gebelik ve Gebelikte Tedabir* stresses physiological factors more than psychological ones as the major causes of miscarriage and pre-term labour. Although this approach diminishes the pressure on mothers, it increases their need for the doctor and medical intervention. Whether it is by disciplining the body, or letting physicians do that for the mother, failing to discipline the body also diminished or eradicated its maternal content.

Of course, gendered assumptions about female nature and the maternal body were inscribed in those arguments. The overriding assumption was that the female body was volatile, especially during pregnancy. The volatility of the maternal body was accompanied and reinforced by the unpredictability and irrationality of the expectant mother according to the presumptions of these books. And it was the doctors' primary role to control and stabilize her volatility.

Craving was emphasized in both books as an explicit indicator of volatility. Although it was not wrong to satisfy their wishes when pregnant women innocently craved sour or sweet things, the manuals emphasize that these wishes could very easily turn to signs of female irrationality, accompanied by the pregnant women's vulnerability and sentimentality. Thus, when craving was not controlled in time, women could be driven to extreme desires, instabilities and perversions. For example, both books argued that there were many women who craved saltpetre, gypsum, rotten meat and even bread dipped into human blood. Moreover, perverted women could crave beating their husbands, or throwing eggs at them, or on the contrary they might ask to be scourged themselves.[42] Such examples implied extreme sexual desires during pregnancy and also equated female sexuality with perversion. Moreover, women were more vulnerable to emotions, such as, sorrow, dread, fury, exasperation, hostility and grudge. And it was argued that such extreme emotions not only made the body volatile but also resulted in miscarriage.[43]

In these manuals doctors were the rational agents of the science of childbirth, whereas women were stigmatized as irrational. Hence, the pregnant woman should put her body under the doctor's scrutiny and to his prescriptions, and not leave pregnancy to the forces of nature. Once the volatility was controlled by the doctor and the husband, women could be the agents of their pregnancy.

Overall, the discourses produced by the prescriptive literature was highly ambivalent. The pregnant woman was sentimental and irrational, but at the same time she continuously had to make judgements. In other words, although these manuals associated woman with irrationality, they, at the same time, assign them reason and the capacity to judge. The women themselves are to decide the appropriate amount of food to eat, make the final decision to go on a long distance trip, or how to entertain themselves. Making judgements and reasoning is the first step of overcoming the volatility and sentimentality of the maternal body, and hence, disciplining it. To state it differently, the advice guides, on the one hand, persistently warned expectant mothers that failing to obey the advice given would put the health and the lives of their children at risk; on the other hand, they left a considerable amount of space for women's individual decision, experience and agency.

Nevertheless, such admonitions were part of the attempt to strip pregnancy of its social content and to medicalize it. As a result of the medical and institutional developments in the nineteenth century, pregnancy started to become a period which should be monitored, checked and controlled by the physicians, and it became less of a stage in the female lifecycle shared by other women. The start of midwifery education in 1842, numerous laws and regulations promoting the entrance of male doctors to obstetrics, the regulation and control of the activities of midwives, the beginning of use of drugs and anaesthesia during childbirth, establishment of the maternity hospital and the proliferation of private maternity clinics, all contributed to medicalizing pregnancy and handing its governance into the hands of male obstetricians. Yet, it would be wrong to conclude that women lost all control over their bodies throughout the course of the nineteenth century. As I have demonstrated, these manuals also assign a substantial degree of agency to expectant mothers. In the end, it was the expectant mother who was to discipline her body and contribute to the health and well-being of her child. In other words, the maternal body of the expectant mother was not merely a site of state intervention or scientific management, but the mother was also seen as being responsible for raising a healthy and disciplined child.

Regulating Pregnancy, Regulating the Offspring

The agency given to women becomes more overt in Halid Ziya's second work on pregnancy and childbirth. After his *Haml u Vaz'ı-Haml*, Halid Ziya produced a second book, *Kanun ve Fenn-i Vilade* (The Laws and Science of Childbirth),[44] again based on and adapted from Auguste Debay's bestselling book *Hygiène et physiologie du mariage*.[45] As with his first book, he selected parts from Debay's volume and put them together through his own interpretation. In this book, it is also possible to find excerpts, summaries and information from several books and treatises by European doctors that are not explicitly or adequately mentioned. Rather than a *mot-a-mot* translation, this work is an adaptation of certain information and ideas regarding the Ottoman context. While *Haml- ü Vaz'ı Haml* is more focused and limits his attention to health care during pregnancy, this second book, *Kanun ve Fenn-i Vilade* (The Laws and Science of Childbirth), is a blend of scientific and popular information, medical generalizations and fantastic exceptions. Nevertheless, the fact that Halid Ziya writing two separate books on the same topic demonstrates that publishing pregnancy manuals had turned into a highly profitable enterprise by the late nineteenth century. Although it is not so easy to know about the number of the copies printed, sold and read, the publication of several books, two of which belong to the very same writer, and a number of popular articles in journals and newspapers demonstrate that this genre attracted popular attention and was indeed sold and read.

Halid Ziya's *Kanun ve Fenn-i Vilade* differs from his previous book as well as the other examples of this genre by its breadth. This popular book does not limit its attention to precautions and discipline during pregnancy but it extends to issues such as infertility and impotence, which were two other important aspects of Ottoman pronatalism. With its fairly broad scope in comparison to other pregnancy manuals available, and its contextualization of proper care during pregnancy with other issues related to the experience of reproduction, *Kanun ve Fenn-i Vilade* offers important insights into the conceptualization of the female body and control of sexuality. This work juxtaposes mythology, antiquarian views, early modern medicine and modern medicine altogether and creates an ahistoric female body and female experience of pregnancy, as if the meanings of these experiences remained unchanged throughout history. However, this conceptualization points out to a political standpoint where Halid Ziya advocates pronatalism as a humanitarian obligation. According to him, 'the real duty of the human beings is to give birth and the most delicate and sacramental goal of humanity is to reproduce'.[46]

Another unique aspect of this book is its extensive use of and reference to tales about pregnancy and childbirth compared to other examples of this genre. For example, one such tale is about a woman who gave birth to fifty-three children: eighteen times she gave birth to one child, five times to twins, three times to triplets; at one pregnancy she gave birth to six, and at another time to seven children.[47] Another example is a certain Elizabeth Pavler, who gave birth to sixteen children. Halid Ziya writes that Pavler and her children were so fertile that she ended up having 114 grandchildren, 228 great grandchildren and 900 great-great grandchildren in her lifetime.[48]

Halid Ziya's exceptional examples are not only about women giving birth to enormous numbers of children; they are also about strange bodies or body parts. For example, he talks about a woman in Rome in 1681 that doctors had observed had more than two breasts. Very strangely, with his wording, she did not only breastfeed with her proper breasts but with her extra one too. According to Halid Ziya, such events were not unseen in Ottoman lands either. In 1827, a doctor, possibly Adrian du Jusyo, had given a report to *Encümen-i Daniş* relating that he had observed a woman with three breasts; two of them were 'normal', while the third was on her groin. What was even stranger is the report that she breastfed her child with this third breast.[49] Finally, he emphasizes functional abnormalities. For example, in the section about menstruation he gives the example of a girl who started to menstruate only eight days after she was born. Another case exemplifying just the opposite is that of a woman who was over forty and with seven children, but had never menstruated. Such strange and exceptional examples, serve to draw a bold line between 'normal' and 'abnormal', 'healthy' and 'sick', 'desirable' and 'morbid', where being normal and healthy was idealized as the desirable.

However, what is at stake is not merely the normality of the parents but the normality of the offspring as well. In order to ensure the health and normality of their children, first of all, the parents should be healthy. In other words, besides being the precondition of fertility, being healthy is also the fundamental requirement of the well-being of the offspring. Halid Ziya asserts that the conditions under which the mother conceived and went through her pregnancy is the most important factor that would affect the physical and moral health of the offspring.[50] Obviously, the better those conditions, the better the physical health and morality of the children.[51] Halid Ziya's emphasis on the impact of the mother's lifestyle before and during pregnancy on the children's health is based on the assumption that the mother's traits are passed to the children, and in order to strengthen his arguments about the inheritance of characteristics, Halid Ziya gives the example of a female dog that was hit by a car and was crippled just before she conceived (*ilkah*); after she gave birth, it was found that seven of her eight puppies were crippled like her.[52]

Although he does not manage to adequately explain the mechanisms of inheritance, the idea that the characteristics of the mother passes to the next generation was still novel when his book was published. Based on this theory, Halid Ziya argues that if harmful habits and situations have a detrimental effect on the mental and physical health of the child, then it is possible to improve the constitution and morality of the child by providing supportive environments during sexual intercourse, conception and pregnancy. This argument was indeed shared by many of the contemporary intellectuals, and constituted the backbone of the disciplinary discourses. Along these lines, Halid Ziya argues that it is most likely that a soldier/musician/sculptor who has sex just after fighting/composing/sculpting would pass on his gifts and abilities to his child.[53] In other words, rather than social factors or the opportunities the family provides, it is a rather simplified cause-and-effect relationship that determines the traits and characteristic of the child.

How can we interpret Halid Ziya's consistent emphasis on the importance of the physical and moral/emotional situation of the mother during pregnancy? When we situate this book within the context of advice books for pregnant women, it advocates disciplining the body and adopting a proper lifestyle during pregnancy, although the type of discipline he counsels is different from the other manuals. The discipline Halid Ziya is advocating is not a medical but rather a moral and behavioural one.

One of the topics that represent his outlook very well is related to the question of whether or not the child will look like something the mother sees during her pregnancy. This question, which Halid Ziya answers affirmatively, is loaded with many assumptions.[54] He asserts that what one sees would determine what one feels. Hence, according to him, it is important to look at beautiful things during pregnancy. Seeing beautiful objects, pictures, scenes would nurture the soul in such as way that the child would benefit from the mother's subsequent serenity. Similarly, experiencing tragic events would negatively affect the character of the child. Halid Ziya devotes a long part to this discussion. He relates another case in which a pregnant woman is attacked by a thief and hurt so badly that she lost consciousness for a while and her head fell sideways for some time. Unfortunately, after the childbirth she discovered that her new born baby could not control her head, which continuously fell sideways and could not be cured. Another pregnant woman who had been scared by a fire had her baby with a red scratch on her face. Even the foetuses of animals are affected by the forces that affect their mothers. For example, if you leave a black piece of fabric into the nest of a pair of white rabbits, Halid Ziya argues, the baby rabbits would be black.[55] Through his examples, Halid Ziya reaches the conclusion that parents who want to ensure the facial beauty and well-proportioned body of their children should make sure to see and observe beautiful landscapes/objects during pregnancy. In short, for Halid Ziya, proper discipline of the maternal body is not limited to eating habits or lifestyles as in the other manuals – here it was sought in the broader environment, aesthetics, and physical and moral standards of the pregnant mother.[56]

The most fundamental question of Halid Ziya's *Kanun ve Fenn-i Vilade* is whether or not something that affects the mother will then affect the foetus, and the purpose of this discussion is to seek to support the relatively novel theory concerning the existence of a link between the mother and the foetus. Halid Ziya underlines and reiterates that those factors that affect the mother would also affect the foetus. Along these lines, Halid Ziya maintains that as the foetus is part of the mother's body (*kısm-ı vücud*), a second body attached to the mother's body, fed by her blood, then while her body feeds and develops the body of the child, so her mind also creates and feeds the mind of the child.[57] Although he cannot always scientifically prove the validity of this theory, the existence of such a cause–effect relationship constitutes the basis of the discourse on the discipline of the pregnant and maternal body. In comparison to his previous book, *Haml u Vaz'-ı Haml*, the essentiality of the discipline of the pregnant body is legitimized in this book.

In Halid Ziya's framework, disciplining the maternal body would also help to manipulate the sex of the child besides her/his health and physical constitution. According to him, through proper diet and adequate lifestyle changes one would cure infertility, choose the sex of the child and secure her/his health and well-being. Thus, discipline is the key to all kinds of reproductive dysfunctions as well as normality and healthiness.

This simplified cause and effect relationship is overt in the discussion of alcoholism. According to Halid Ziya, alcoholism has a highly negative affect on the health and constitution of the children. He argues that the children of the parents who have the habit of drinking are more prone to become alcoholics and he continues with examples to support this view. He details the story of a doctor who cured two brothers who were both alcoholics. Upon interrogating their mother, he found out – to no surprise, Halid Ziya notes – that she was drunk at the time of conception.[58] Another similar example is that of an alcoholic musician whose daughters and sons alike had either mental or physical handicaps as a result of their father's poor traits.[59] Halid Ziya also gives examples from history to support his claim and he cites that Diogenes had once said to a shapeless young man 'your father must have been very drunk when your mother generated you (*hasıl etmek*)'. He also refers to Plutarch who he claims to have said that one would not be able to harvest crops if he sows soil in a drunken state.[60] According to Halid Ziya, such examples support the link between drunkenness and unhealthiness.

However, given the limitations of contemporary knowledge on the rules and mechanisms of heredity, both Halid Ziya and his sources were rather unclear about the connections between the traits of the mother and the child. The debate on alcoholism offers us a peculiar opportunity to examine the thin line between pronatalism and eugenics. Halid Ziya comes to the conclusion that those with negative characteristics such as alcoholism should not allowed to reproduce. According to him, in order to deserve to be parent one should continuously develop positive traits through appropriate lifestyle choices and diet. Eugenicist ideas were more widely debated by Ottoman intellectuals after the turn of the century and especially in the political context of the Second Constitutional period.

The Thin Line between Pronatalism and Eugenics: Pregnancy Manuals and the Idea of Good Birth

The conceptualization of the female body as a 'maternal body' and the promotion of medical discipline during pregnancy were receiving a wider audience as the century closed and as Ottoman pronatalism was consolidated. Even one of the most profit- oriented figures of Ottoman print culture, Seyyid Mehmed Tahir Bey, published an advice book for pregnant women, which tellingly demonstrates the attention this genre received by the intellectuals and the literate public. Seyyid Mehmed Tahir was a prolific writer and publisher, who published quite a large number of books and periodicals targeting women, and written by women. He was the owner of the newspapers *Malumat* (Information) and *Servet* (Fortune), as well as the *İtimat* (Reliability) printing houses.[61] Seyyid Mehmed Tahir had published extensively on topics such as women's liberation, the equality of men and women, and the relations between men and women. However, his motivation was far from the emancipation of women, instead serving profit and self-interest.[62] Thus, Seyyid Mehmed Tahir's attentiveness of issues related to pregnancy and childbirth shows that texts instructing pregnant women were receiving an increasing audience and readership, and becoming quite popular in the context of late nineteenth early twentieth-century anxieties of depopulation. And topics related to women such as marriage, sexuality, women's liberation and health started to appear more and more in print targeted at Ottoman women as well.[63]

The pregnancy manual prepared and published by Seyyid Mehmed Tahir, *Vaz'ı Haml: İbtia-ı Hamil, Kabilenin Vazifesi, Cenin* (Childbirth: The Beginning of Pregnancy, the Duties of the Midwife, Embryo and Fetus) is quite a short book of twenty-nine pages. This book is based on French and German sources that Seyyid Mehmed Tahir does not identify clearly, but we understand that this is mostly translation and summary of several books on the topic. Seyyid Mehmed Tahir clearly saw that advice literature on pregnancy and child care was becoming a profitable field, since he announced that he would be publishing several other books on the topic. Although it seems that he never published the successive works, he promised to cover issues such as false pregnancy, the determination of the sex of the baby, the changes in the body during pregnancy, the determination of the date of birth and hygiene during pregnancy.

Similar to the other books on this topic, the main problem of Seyyid Mehmed Tahir's *Vaz'ı Haml* is the population question and the threat of depopulation on the Ottoman lands. At the very opening, Seyyid Mehmed Tahir notes that European cultures attach great value to the increase of population, and the Ottomans share this concern as can be testified by the *Quran* and other sacred writings. According to him, the religion Islam allowed polygamy in order to promote population growth. However, Seyyid Mehmed Tahir laments that the religious and humanitarian duty to produce a good number of offspring was largely disregarded in the Ottoman society despite the proclivities of Islam. He despises that most of his contemporaries have at most two children, while in the past men used to have twenty to thirty. He also makes a connection between the number of children a man has and the health and well-being of those children, and reaches the conclusion that the higher the number of children in a family, the healthier they are. According to him, the biggest menace threatening the Ottoman society is not only the low birth rates, but also the poor health and constitution of those born.[64] Seyyid Mehmed Tahir, who followed contemporary social issues and debates very closely, was aware of the existence of the same fears of depopulation in Europe as he compares the Ottoman case with the situation in France and Germany.[65]

Seyyid Mehmed Tahir's reasons for slow birth rates hark back to the discourses on debauchery as the main cause of abortion. According to him, one of the main reasons why women avoid giving birth is their frailty, and weakness, as well as their tendency towards make-up, dress and entertainments at night; he subscribes to the idea that Ottoman women cannot reject the pleasures of night life, and fearing that they would be missing sleep once they have children, they avoid pregnancy. It is mostly the poor families according to him who have larger number of children, but since they lack the resources to raise well mannered children, their children do not benefit the well-being of the Ottoman country but instead act as a burden to it.[66] Due to the importance of the magnitude and the well-being of the population, Seyyid Mehmed Tahir believes, couples should be checked before marriage and those who are not in good health ought to be banned from marriage. However, he laments, this important duty is virtually out of practice in the Ottoman country.[67] In his work, pronatalism is not merely about giving birth to more children and population increase. The well-being of those born, their characteristics and the overall qualities of the population, are important issues to be considered in relation to the political and economic exigencies of the Ottoman country; especially the need for healthier and wealthier generations and underlined boldly.

Seyyid Mehmed Tahir's mode of thinking is stereotypical of the Ottoman pronatalists' comprehension of the population problem. The eugenic ideas he was loudly expressing were indeed becoming popular on Ottoman lands.[68] After the turn of the century, especially in the context of the Second Constitutional Period, eugenic and social-Darwinist ideas were debated widely and expressively among the Ottoman intellectuals.[69] We can see similar ideas expressed in more refined ways in Besim Ömer's translation of Auguste Debay's *Sıhhatnüma-yı İzdivac: Evleneceklerle Müteehhil ve Mücerred Bulunanlara Nasihat* (The Ways for Healthy Marriage: Advice for the Married, the Single and those Who Would Marry),[70] and his *Fen ve İzdivac: Evlenebilecekler ve Evlenemeyecekler* (Science and Marriage: Those Who Could and Could Not Marry).[71] Besim Ömer, as discussed above, was one of the most ardent supporters of Ottoman and then later early Republican pronatalism. His latter books express pronatalist and eugenic ideas more explicitly. However, in the period under scrutiny in this work, it is only possible to find vague hints of what was to come.

When we turn back to Seyyid Mehmed Tahir, similar to the other pregnancy manuals, he comprehends women as the producers of the population. The goal he serves through publishing this pregnancy manual is to advise and to manipulate Ottoman women to produce more and healthier children. Along these lines, he first informed women about the process of childbirth and then advised them not to wear weird dresses during pregnancy and to obey the rules of hygiene and medicine.[72] Although he does not make clear what he means by referring to 'weird dress', the tone of his writings is familiar to us from the previous pregnancy manuals. What Seyyid Mehmed Tahir tries to advocate in the end is the disciplinary discourses expressed in Besim Ömer's and Halid Ziya's advice books. This book also reiterates that bodily discipline is the precondition of morality and virtue (*maneviyye* and *ahlakiyye*).[73] Disciplining the female body means disciplining the younger and forthcoming generations of children and hence humanity. Similar to Besim Ömer, Tahir repeats that the health and bodily strength of the child depends on that of the mother as well as on her efforts and precautions to maintain her child's health.[74] The happiness of the family entails the bodily, moral and spiritual discipline of the mother more than anything else. It is not surprising to read Seyyid Mehmed Tahir writing that disciplining the female body is a humanitarian duty, and should be accomplished first by disciplining young girls.[75] According to him, once the body of a young girl is disciplined, this humanitarian goal is accomplished almost by eighty per cent.[76]

The pronatalist context within which advice literature about health care during pregnancy emerged also constituted a prolific background for the emergence of discourses on girlhood.[77] The normative literature of pregnancy made a bold emphasis on the discipline of young girls; hence it is not surprising to see the proliferation of advice literature about disciplining girls. According to the pronatalists, the discipline of girls was the first step of the process to raise physically and morally healthy generations. Advice books targeting young girls and advocating and counselling their discipline is hence a fruitful field of advice literature in that period.[78]

The prescriptive books on the discipline of girls targeted the mothers of girls more than the young girls themselves, and advised them of the best ways to raise their daughters and to prepare them for marriage and motherhood. Advice books for young girls comprise a great variety of topics from childhood to marriage and childbirth. We can find advice about how to soothe small children to how to dress them, the physical and psychological changes during adolescence, the female physiology, menstruation, sexuality, masturbation, pregnancy and last but not the least, childbirth. All kinds of information from diet to dress were included in such books. But the most significant of all advice given is related to sexual education of the girls. Although the purpose of this education is to prepare girls for marriage, these books do feel the need to note that a girl who lacked such an education would not be aware of the importance of avoiding any sexual activity prior to marriage.

As previously mentioned, these books also refer to mothers of young girls and remind them of the importance of disciplining their daughters in terms of their physical, mental and moral health. Ignoring such discipline might lead to grave and irreversible mistakes. The knowledge about sexuality would prepare young girls for marriage and eventually motherhood. Here we can also talk about the invention of girlhood as a moral category.[79]

Seyyid Mehmed Tahir's book gives more space to ideals and norms compared to actual rules and advice. Presumably because he had in mind to publish more books and manuals on this issue, he expressed mostly his ideas rather than formulating practical, daily advice for pregnant women. This pregnancy manual again points out the need to medicalize pregnancy and childbirth. Seyyid Mehmed Tahir underlines the necessity to see a doctor or a midwife (here he uses the term doctor-midwife (*ebe-doktor*), which means male midwife) during pregnancy. He notes that although pregnancy is not a sickness or illness, it is a time when the female body becomes more vulnerable to all kind of diseases.[80] He suggests that the kidneys and the liver especially become vulnerable during pregnancy and hence he advises pregnant women to have a doctor's or a midwife's check-up during this period. A doctor's or a midwife's check-up in the eighth month of pregnancy would also provide knowledge about the position of the baby. Here, Seyyid Mehmed Tahir notes that if the foetus is positioned correctly, the birth will not be too difficult, but in cases of breech deliveries or when the position of the foetus is not right, unless a doctor (who is naturally male) or a male midwife handles the operation and turns the foetus inside the uterus, the parturition would be very dangerous and the baby's life would be at risk.[81]

As stereotypical of this genre, the second part of this book is spared for the signs of pregnancy. Here we have hints about the goal and the audience of this book, as well. Seyyid Mehmed Tahir notes that most of the newly married young women are embarrassed to see and to be seen by a doctor. As a result they avoid referring to a doctor, most of the time. However, since they also lack experience, in many cases they mistakenly diagnose themselves without the guidance of their doctors. He writes that it is not rare for newly married young women to believe that they are pregnant and become disappointed when they find out they are not.[82] However, these women also sometimes fail to recognize their pregnancies and hence fail to take the necessary precautions. As a result, he argues, many such women miscarry and are sometimes left maimed or barren. In this way, Seyyid Mehmed Tahir warns young mothers that their embarrassment and avoidance of doctor's check-ups may deprive them from future pregnancy and children.

By late century, pregnancy turned into a site of Ottoman pronatalism and the politics of the female body. Discourses on the discipline during pregnancy were not monolithic and fixed, however. The earlier approaches about care during pregnancy advocated a more medical discipline of female body. As different voices were raised the nature of the prescriptions also started to change. The pregnancy manuals offer us important clues about Ottoman pronatalists' conceptions of female reproduction and femininity. Moreover, they are an important site within which early eugenic ideas were expressed. In order to be able to talk about the Social Darwinist and eugenic ideas within an Ottoman context, we should wait the Second Constitutional period. However, the late Tanzimat period also offers some hints regarding the idea of good birth and good breading as conceived by Ottoman intellectuals.

The pronatalist policies of the late nineteenth century were not only interested in the quantity of the population as before, but paid increasing attention to its quality. Therefore, the Ottoman government and intellectuals not only encouraged women to bear larger numbers of children, but also, for the first time, took the health and wellness of these children as important goals. The pregnancy manuals also emphasized the importance of the well-being of the population and played important roles in defining the corresponding criteria. Health, according to the manuals, was not a natural characteristic, but could be achieved by disciplining the body. The population the government sought had to be strong, active and brave, which could be bred only by raising children scientifically. And that could be achieved, if and only if, a similar medical and scientific approach was applied to all stages covering before, during and after childbirth. Finally, only a decade later, Ottoman intellectuals started to express the idea that who should reproduce was also an important issue, and they increasingly emphasized the notion that that the Ottoman country needed the reproduction of people who were able to raise healthy, well-built and educated children. They called upon those families who were able to provide such qualities to their offspring to give birth to more children, and these families were indeed the targeted audience of the advice literature on pregnancy.

5 INFERTILITY AS A PUBLIC PROBLEM

> validelikten mahrum kalmış olmak acısı; daima zehirnak yerden katre ile damlayan bir cerehadır. Zan olunur ki kudret katre kadınların sine-i revhına boş kalmağa tahammül edemeyen bir beşik koymuştur.[1]
>
> (Being deprived of motherhood is like pus dripping drop by drop from the poisoned place. One feels it as if God had placed an empty cradle that cannot bear being empty to the lap of women.)

The final element of Ottoman pronatalism examined here is the medical and popular discourses on infertility. As I have mentioned throughout this book, Ottoman political power and the medical elites devoted most of their energy to increasing the birth rates and decreasing maternal and infant death rates, and they focused on encouraging women to give birth to more children. However, most of the policies implemented were based on the assumption that women already wanted to have children and that they were able to do so. What was left out of the scope of pronatalist policies until late century was the problem of infertility.

As discussed in the previous chapters, the fate of the population and the demographic anxieties were shaped by broader political contentions. By the end of the century, in the Ottoman lands, reproduction and female sexuality had turned into political phenomena, and they were no longer conceived as merely biological functions. This concern with the population was not only a matter of numbers, however. Besides being an arena of wider political controversies, the demographic question was gendered, too, where femininity was defined in relation to the ability to reproduce. Within this context, women's experiences of reproduction were classified, manipulated and judged by the political actors. Yet, Ottoman pronatalism did not remain fixed throughout the century. As the nature of Ottoman pronatalism was changing parallel to social and intellectual shifts, a final issue that remained overlooked, started to receive attention, and the problem of infertility as a medical problem emerged as another factor curtailing population growth. In other words, towards the end of the nineteenth century, Ottoman intellectuals turned their attention to a hitherto overlooked arena of female reproduction. While the regulation of midwifery, bans on abortion and medical encroachment upon pregnancy and childbirth were targeting female experiences of childbirth, they were all concerned with women who experienced pregnancy, gave birth or terminated the pregnancy for their own reasons. The pronatalists had assumed that all women were able to give birth and concentrated their energies on the ways to increase their fecundity. However, there were also women who remained childless despite their desire to have children, and medical elites and intellectuals redefined infertility as a problem hindering their pronatalist goals. Part of the former inattentiveness lay in the lack of contemporary medical knowledge regarding infertility solutions. As the close of the century approached, contemporary levels of the obstetrical/ gynaecological knowledge started to explain, diagnose and cure at least some cases of infertility, which made infertility an area of pronatalist battle.

Infertility or the involuntary childlessness is the focus of the final chapter of this work and Ottoman pronatalism. The control and manipulation of female sexuality and women's bodies was finally framed with the discussion and problematization of infertility. Examination of the debates on infertility is important first for a final consideration of the issue of women's agency in Ottoman society. In the last decades of the nineteenth century, Ottoman pronatalism and issues related to fertility increasingly made their appearance in Ottoman publishing. Books and journal and newspaper articles advocating pronatalist ideals directly and indirectly gained prominence as the Ottoman print culture developed and started to target popular audience beside the elites. The books on male and female infertility should be contextualized with regard to the flourishing of advice books on all kinds of topics including but not limited to family, marriage, hygiene and childcare. Books advising married women, married men, young girls, single men and couples emerged in this period.[2] Prescriptive literature also appealed to married couples and to those who were intending to get married.[3] The normative literature also discussed who should get married and who should not.[4] Finally, more popular books dealing with the question of determining the sex of children can also be located within that genre.[5]

The normative literature played an important function in popularizing pronatalist ideals as well as medical knowledge. As was the case for pregnancy manuals, we can find reprints or later additions of the advice books about marriage, which demonstrates that these advice books were sold and read relatively widely despite the low literacy level in Ottoman society. It is usually argued that the appearance of women's issues on Ottoman newspapers and journals, as well as the emergence of women's journals should be taken as a signpost of women's emancipation.[6] However, it is not so easy to reach to the same conclusion when examining the literature on infertility. Those books, on the one hand, challenge the traditional views on marriage and the relations between men and women, and do advocate unconventional ideas as a result. On the other hand, however, it is controversial that the role assigned to women is emancipatory. In relation to the pronatalist goals, by their almost uncritical advocacy of this political target, the normative literature placed women in the role of mothers and producers of children almost exclusively. By its subscription of the pronatalist ideals, the literature on infertility either posited women as patients to be cured by the medical doctors, or as the victims of their wrongdoings.

The analysis of the debates and discourses on infertility and impotence is insightful, secondly, for bringing in the question of male body. While the other venues of Ottoman pronatalism targeted the female body solely, reproductive disabilities and dysfunctions also concerned the male body. Besides the female body and female sexuality, male sexual dysfunctions were to be regulated as part of the national, humanitarian and political duties according to the pronatalists. Although this chapter limits its attention to the debates on female infertility, it touches upon male infertility and impotence when necessary. In late nineteenth century and early twentieth century, it is possible to find a good number of books discussing the reasons and possible remedies of impotence.[7] These books underlined that impotence and infertility were two different issues. While this literature saw impotence as a problem that could be cured easily through appropriate precautions and remedies, it found it more difficult to cure female infertility. Hence, the books on impotence outnumbered the books on female infertility. Yet, the examination of debates on infertility help us to further refine our analysis of Ottoman pronatalism.

Finally, infertility, the inability to conceive and/or to give birth is a topic that involves assumptions about the female body more than the previous topics examined in this research. The analysis of Ottoman pronatalism demonstrates that the boundaries of the female body were not fixed and stable but rather vague. Indeed, the line between the individual body and the social body is also not clear. The discussion in this chapter demonstrates strongly that sexuality, impregnation and venereal health were not biological/physiological issues but rather political topics. Thus, the examination of the medical and normative literature on infertility offer rich insights into how the personal and social blended into each other in the particular context of nineteenth-century Ottoman pronatalism. It shows us that the body is never merely personal and intimate, but it is in fact a battlefield of broader political contentions and goals. The analysis of the Ottoman policies of reproduction and female sexuality force us to reconsider the nature of the intimate and the political. While the examination of the intimate tells us a lot about the public, the public fulfils itself through its control and manipulation of the intimate.

Infertility and the Infertile: Illness or Punishment? Patient or Victim?

Discourses on fertility became conspicuous towards the end of the century. Increasing birth rates was a national duty according to Ottoman intellectuals and medical elites. However, some women were not able to contribute to this valuable duty for different reasons. The literature on infertility conceived the problem of infertility on different bases, and proposed different cures or solutions, as a result. According to some writers, infertility was predominantly a physiological or a medical problem and hence should be cured by a medical expert. For others, it was the outcome of a personal or behavioural pathology. Some saw it as a factor curbing happiness in marriage; others believed that infertility is provoked by the problems in marriage. Some writers heralded that the problem of infertility would be erased thanks to novel medical developments, such as 'artificial fertilization'; others said that it would take time for these medical technologies to develop and produce fruitful results. In sum, the approaches towards infertility were not monolithic, and the reasons and cures of infertility were tightly linked to the political agendas of its stakeholders.

Although many different intellectual figures devoted their energy to discuss and cure infertility, Besim Ömer was again the pioneer, writing a book directly on this topic. As discussed elaborately in the previous chapters, Besim Ömer was, indeed, a major advocate and protagonist of Ottoman and later early Republican pronatalism. Besides his intensive work on pregnancy, childbirth and midwifery, he wrote about infertility both directly and indirectly. While he touched upon this issue in his works on different topics, he wrote a medical monograph, *Ukum ve Ananet* (Infertility and Impotence), in 1890/1, and examined the reasons and cures of infertility. In this work, he directly addressed the problem of infertility and impotence, and discussed in quite a detailed way the physiological, medical, and social causes of the reproductive dysfunctions. Although the title promised to cover both problems, the major part of the book was devoted to female infertility rather than male impotence.[8]

Since *Ukum ve Ananet* deals both with infertility and impotence, Besim Ömer at the very beginning makes a distinction between the two. According to him, infertility is the inability to reproduce whereas impotence is the inability to get involved in sexual intercourse.[9] *Ukum ve Ananet* consists of nine chapters. In the first chapter, Besim Ömer defines his problem and gives general information. In the second chapter, he talks about women's diseases that may lead to infertility, their reasons, and their remedies. The third and forth chapters are about the problems that affect the uterus and lead to infertility. Besim Ömer discusses very elaborately the problems with the structure of the uterus, and the most common deformations in its shape, as well as their surgical solutions. The fifth chapter is devoted to menstruation and ovulation and to their link with fertility. In the sixth chapter, Besim Ömer comes to psychological, behavioural and/or social factors that may lead to infertility, and talks about nymphomania, excessive sexual activity, vaginismus, obesity and the disproportion of the physical characteristics of the couple such as their weight and length. Chapter seven is relatively a short one, which is partly a summary; and in the eighth chapter, Besim Ömer talks about the importance of medical treatment, rest and hygiene to cure infertility. Here it is significant that he also underlines the importance of hygiene not only for the patients but for the doctors as well. Although the title promises to cover impotence besides infertility, this topic is handled only in the ninth and final chapter.

Besim Ömer's book is quite medical compared to the other examples of the literature about infertility. Yet the main frame of his work is devoted to the most usual and frequent cases. Accordingly, at the very beginning, Besim Ömer tells that he is writing *Ukum ve Ananet* to help couples who fail to have children, and mentions he would be focusing on the most common causes of infertility. This book emphasizes those situations that are generally easier to cure, and unique and exceptional cases are left apart with the recommendation of a doctor's treatment.[10] One of Besim Ömer's major goals was to familiarize lay audience with medical knowledge and the benefits of modern medicine, and he accordingly used a literary style that could be followed and digested without much difficulty. In his popular works, he positioned folk practices of medicine and modern medicine as oppositional pairs, and while he was denigrating the former, glorified the latter. In his work on infertility, as well, he denigrated the role of midwives to cure infertility. He also harshly criticized the use of folk practices such as herbs, amulets, or prayers, and emphasized over and over that one should consult a doctor when confronted with infertility problems.

Besim Ömer starts his debate on infertility with a brief summary of his ideas on the importance of population. His emphasis on the importance of hospitals at the introduction gives the clues of the medicalization approach that he would be defending throughout the book. Here, he underlines that as part of the goal to increase Ottoman population, it is vital to establish specialized hospitals including maternity clinics that would serve poor and lonely (*acize*) women and provide them a safe environment to give child birth.[11]

As expressed in his other books, as well, childlessness, the inability to give birth, is the worst of all the calamities a woman could experience, according to Besim Ömer. With his own words, childlessness is 'like a wound that incessantly bleeds to intoxicate and reinjure itself'. This suffering was so great; it was as if fate had placed a cradle on women's laps that could not put up with being empty.[12] It is not surprising that the choice not to give birth was completely out of question in this framework. According to Besim Ömer, only immoral women tried to escape their duty to raise children, and these women could not even be accepted as women. In the cases where they did conceive, such women tried to murder their babies by abortion. Besim Ömer in his popular and medical works alike assumes a direct connection between morality and reproduction. Moral women give birth to children and discipline both their bodies and their children's bodies as an indication of their morality, whereas immoral women fail to do so.

In his *Ukm ve Ananet*, Besim Ömer gives very detailed descriptions of female pathologies resulting in the inability to conceive and/or in ability to continue a fertile pregnancy. According to him infertility may have physiological, social, and psychological causes and hence should be treated accordingly under the control of a physician. One of the most common reasons of infertility is vaginal/uterus infections.[13] Besim Ömer even gives statistics and tells that ten or twelve of every twenty women, who seek medical help for infertility, suffer such infections.[14] The defections of the uterus are also among the medical causes of infertility and discussed in detail in the third part of the book. He mentions that many problems with the uterus can only be cured by surgical means. However, we should note that Besim Ömer does not support the execution of surgical operation in most cases in order not to risk the life of the mother. Such operations endanger the life of the woman and hence should be avoided. According to him, when the operation is not conducted, that woman will not have any children, but when it is conducted, her life would be risked. He compares the life of a woman with the life of unborn children and reaches the conclusion that their life cannot be risked.[15] Only in cases when the medical and surgical means that do not risk the life of the woman are available, he says, such operations should be conducted.

Some of the factors that contribute to fertility are age, lifestyle, diet, climate, ethnicity (*kavmiyyet*), tells Besim Ömer. The best age recommended to give birth and to have children is between twenty and thirty. A difference more than twenty years of age between the couples would produce infertile results and most probably childlessness according to him. The climate is also important, Besim Ömer says, and icy and cold northern climates are not suitable for reproduction whereas fertility rates increases as one move toward the south. The most important factor to increase fecundity and to be able to give birth to numerous children is to be healthy. The health of the genitals is seen as utmost important, in this respect.

Besim Ömer, very elaborately discusses menstruation, ovulation, function of the ovaries, the link between menstruation and conception in relation to fertility. Despite the technical and medical aspect of the topic, Besim Ömer tries to simplify his presentation through examples from the nature. He also notes that although menstruation and the proper functioning of the ovaries are the precondition of fertility, they do not always guarantee conception. Referring to nature he says that, 'It is very natural that not all the trees which have flowers give fruit eventually'.[16] He also writes, 'We observe that some older trees in our gardens flower and salute spring with their scents, they wither away with the first breeze. Such flowers are their last farewell, the kisses of secession.'[17]

Ukum ve Ananet talks about the latest medical approaches to infertility. It elaborately describes its reasons and cures. The physiology of reproduction was increasingly defined within the domain of medical science.[18] As opposed to the approach of the other extant books about infertility which see this problem as a moral punishment, Besim Ömer's work handles it not as a punishment but as a medical situation. As such it has a rather progressive approach which encourages the couples to consult a doctor and search for treatments. Yet, the medicalization of infertility constructed the doctor and the patient in quite a hierarchical relationship where the patient was submissive to the doctor. Besim Ömer condemns the traditional view that sees the women alone responsible – even handicapped – for infertility, emphasizes that the men do also have their share in involuntary childlessness, and states that couples should search solutions together. He sees husbands as responsible for infertility as well, and he deviates from the mainstream literature by not constructing women as handicapped victims. Yet, the medicalization approach does not give full space to female agency. The infertile is a patient to be cured by the doctor. She is supposed to have pathologies that were to be diagnosed, classified, and controlled by the physician. As such, she is constructed as submissive to the doctors. While the pregnant has some agency pending upon her *mot-a-mot* following of the principles as prescribed by the doctor, the infertile is not an agent but a pathological body. According to Besim Ömer, infertility is a problem to be handled by the medical experts. Unless its causes are searched and diagnosed by the doctors, it is not easy, even possible to cure infertility. Rather than folk beliefs, amulets, prayers, the couples need medical diagnose as well as a doctor's prescription to overcome infertility. Thus, infertility is medicalized by Besim Ömer. By medicalization, I mean that the infertile is conceptualized as a patient in this perspective. In order to cure this illness, she should be checked by a doctor and then follow his advice and prescriptions. Thus, she is subject to the doctor-patient relationship, in which the rules are defined by the doctor and followed by the patient.[19]

Indeed, folk practices have always been helpful to cure infertility. There have been many traditional remedies that were believed to cure infertility or to provoke fertility.[20] Midwives also have played important roles to cure infertility throughout history. In Besim Ömer's frame, unfortunately, there is no reference to the midwives. But between the lines, he stringently opposes the use of magic or sorcery to cure infertility, and condemns the folk practices of midwifery as another form of sorcery. He insists that the causes of infertility either come from birth or caused later as a result of age, character, medical conditions. The treatment of fertility mostly requires medical means and a doctor's supervision.

Yet, the level of medical knowledge on the reasons and cures of infertility led Besim Ömer to leave an open space to some fortuities as an explanation of some evens that he could not well justify rationally otherwise, despite his insistence on medical science. A case experience by Paju, a prominent French obstetrician, and discussed by Besim Ömer is significant to show the limitations of the medicalization paradigm, in this respect.[21] Paju, in Besim Ömer's account tells that he was consulted by an aristocratic woman who had never experienced a pregnancy but who desires a lot to have a child. She tells him that she was checked by prominent women's doctors in different European capitals, but with the exception of one doctor, Skanzoni, who was again one another highly prominent contemporary obstetrician/gynaecologist, she was told that her uterus is defected and not fit for pregnancy. Paju, upon his check sees that her uterus is located below her cervix, and bended on its own. However, when he learns that her periods are regular and not painful concludes that it is difficult but not impossible for her to become pregnant. After a few months, the same woman calls him saying that she felt a very strong pain in her abdomen. Paju finds out that her uterus had turned into its normal shape and she is pregnant just as he had foreseen, and concludes that the pain must be derived from the sudden straightening of her uterus. He also notes that she had given birth to a healthy baby, but her uterus turned into its bended shape a while after the parturition.[22] Leaving apart the curious question whether this case is medically possible or not, it is significant that Besim Ömer finds this event possible and devotes a long section to it. Despite the developments in the fields of gynaecology and obstetrics, the level of medical knowledge was still limited when it came to infertility. When he could not explain the case adequately, he took his source, Paju, as an authority.

As could be observed in this case, Besim Ömer's paradigm is not without its gaps. Although in many places, the infertile is a patient to be checked, cured by the doctor, it is significant that he assigns an important degree of agency to the infertile couple when it comes to disciplining their routines. For example, in the cases when the uterus is bended or inclined to one side, Besim Ömer advises the husband to lean his wife to the opposite side during sexual intercourse in order to increase fertility.[23] The cure is easy in some cases. For a woman whose uterus in bended forward, he advises retreating from going to the toilet and doing this just before sexual intercourse. In the opposite case, when the uterus bended backward, rather than emptying the bladder, the woman should keep it full by following a diet that would lead to constipation.[24] This view gives agency both to the women and the couple. Although the infertile is a patient, she can contribute to her therapy.

Although nineteenth century anxieties of depopulation turned infertility a hot topic of public debate there were more than one approach toward the reasons, treatments and harms of infertility. As infertility became a political problem, the ways it was handled started increasingly to reflect the political standpoints and agendas of its debaters.

Another popular work that deals with the female inability to give birth is the work translated by Avanzade Süleyman, *Mesail-i Mühimme-i Hayatiye ve Sıhhiyeden Kısır Kadınlar* (Important Problems about Life and Health: Infertile Women).[25] Avanzade Süleyman[26] has translated this book from a French source on the same topic. Rather than being a *mot-a-mot* or exact translation, it is an adaptation where he took some parts of the original source and left out some others in accordance with his aims and approaches, and without acknowledging the author and name of his source. In late nineteenth and early twentieth century such adaptations were quite frequent in Ottoman print culture. Avanzade Süleyman also made a later adaptation of a similar kind on impotence *Adem-i İktidar* (Impotence).[27] Although *Mesail-i Mühimme-i Hayatiye ve Sıhhiyeden Kısır Kadınlar* promises to cover female infertility, this book is rather limited to artificial fertilization (*ilkah-ı suni*), which was a novel, yet rather an unreliable medical technology back then. Still, this book is quite a unique source to analyze Ottoman pronatalism and the discourses on infertility, or involuntary childlessness.

Avanzade Süleyman's book is relatively a short one and it is rather unfocused with its frequent shift between female infertility and male infertility. The language used evokes many hidden and discrete references to sexuality, especially when compared to Besim Ömer's book, which is more medical and disciplinary. However, the publication of such popular books demonstrates the success of Ottoman pronatalism. Towards the end of the century, the debate about reproduction, female sexuality, and the means to raise population through the manipulation of reproduction has been more or less consolidated. The vocabulary and discourses used in this genre assume a certain definition of population. Especially in popular books there is no open reference to any specific *millet*, ethnic or religious group. Since most of the examples are taken directly from books published in French and hence reconstruct the experiences of women and men with infertility problems in Europe, it is hard to have a glimpse of local experiences and practices. *Mesail-i Mühimmeden Kısır Kadınlar*, for example, builds upon many real cases. However, these cases have been unexceptionally taken from the accounts, reports, and memoirs of European and sometimes American doctors. The short note on the cover of the book reminds that the initial emphasis on '*tenperverlik*' (debauchery) is still valid in some contexts. This note tells that 'although infertility/barrenness protects the beauty of the body, it is a quality that does not contribute to humanity'.[28]

The debates on infertility diverge from the previous pronatalist policies that I have examined by targeting a male audience and problematizing the male body. The professionalization of midwifery, bans on abortion and the medicalization of pregnancy and childbirth were prominently directed to controlling the female body and sexuality. However, infertility was not only a sexual dysfunction waiting women but it was also a problem experienced by men. When the male body was concerned the approaches usually made a distinction between infertility and impotence.

Halid Ziya's *Kanun ve Fenn-i Vilade*, is one of the rare books that addressed male audience explicitly.[29] Although this book is similar in its approach and premises to his previous work, it is different than it by targeting male audience besides female. In fact, this book is the only available example of this genre targeting explicitly male audience. As such, it offers us a unique opportunity to see those marginal areas where Ottoman pronatalist policies refer to the male population as their audience. At the opening, Halid Ziya mentions that this book tries to target men and women who want to have children, who are getting prepared to become fathers and mothers. Pronatalist assumptions are implicit in this book, too, and although he mostly uses such ideas implicitly, only at the start he mentions that the real duty of the human beings is to give birth, and the most delicate and sacramental duty of humanity is reproduction.[30]

Halid Ziya uses the metaphor of garden and tree frequently to describe infertility similar to Avanzade Süleyman. *Mesail-i Mühimmeden Kısır Kadınlar*, for instance, tells on its cover page that 'a barren woman is like a wild tree. Both have to be grafted and ameliorated for breeding'. The term 'to be grafted' (*aşılanmak*) is used frequently to refer to the means of curing and impregnating infertile women.[31] Moreover, in order to denote children, both books use the term '*semere*', which can be translated as fruit, harvest or crop.

Avanzade Süleyman asserts that the Holly Book, the book of humanity and the book of nature all call for marriage, which is the alliance of men and women, and all order humans to produce offspring and carry on their descent. He claims that all the different divine laws converge when it comes to marriage. According to him, they all order the same, which is to marry and to reproduce. He calls this universal command the law of marriage, and denotes this as the book of marriage.[32]

In Avanzade Süleyman's work, the animal and plant species are frequently used as metaphors. He says that all the living beings on earth, the animals and the plants come together, fertilize, and produce offspring. To him, it is only the stones that do not want to reproduce.[33] Human beings accordingly should come together and reproduce. It is the nature which dictates a woman and a man to love each other. However, in the nature love is never merely a unification of physical bodies, but nature wants the produce of love, as well. According to Avanzade Süleyman, when the couples fail to have a child, when they fail to produce offspring, an outcome, a produce, they would separate eventually.[34] No marriage can survive without producing an outcome which is the child, he asserts. Besim Ömer also agrees that a childless couple would either fight every day, or be dragged to an ultimate silence and unhappiness.[35] According to the Ottoman intellectuals, having a child is natural law, social necessity, and personal source of happiness, whereas childlessness is a tragedy.

According to Besim Ömer the diagnosing the reasons of impotence and curing it lies in medical factors. Avanzade's approach is different, however. Although he asserts this latently, it is always the women that should be blamed for fertility. However, luckily, there is a novel but almost certain remedy, which is artificial fertilization. Avanzade Süleyman's book describes this novelty, the methods and the procedure of its practice. He also exemplifies it with real case stories as observed by contemporary European doctors.

One of the issues that come out of this book is the compatibility of this novel method with religious duties and principles. Avanzade tells that the sperm of the husband is placed into the womb of his wife through a small pipe. Therefore, there is no reason to fear immorality, and avoid such a procedure.[36] When a person cannot be fed because of a problem in her throat, the doctors feed her through a catheter, similarly, Avanzade Süleyman tells, when a couple have sexual intercourse but fail to have a child, the fresh sperm of the husband is transferred to the wife's womb through a catheter.[37] He also tells that in Ottoman society most vaginal operations are not redeemed as moral or vice, and hence asserts that there is no reason to avoid artificial fertilization. In the cases when the couple has been married longer than two years but failed to have a child, it would be legitimate for the couple to try this method.[38]

This book also differs profoundly from Besim Ömer's in terms of the agency it attests to ordinary couples. At the end of the book, Avanzade Süleyman tells that a man who is familiar with the rules of science and has some manual dexterity, and also has some knowledge about female genital anatomy can fertilize his wife without any need to doctor.[39] Although reference to science and medicine is important, the agency is not limited to medical doctors. Besim Ömer also talks about artificial fertilization like Avanzade Süleyman.[40] After describing the procedure, he advocates its importance. Yet, he is more critical of its results, and suffices to announcing it.

Although Ottoman intellectuals agreed that infertility was a hidden menace causing depopulation, their approaches to the reasons and remedies of infertility were different. Besides approaches medicalizing infertility, we can talk about views that see it as a stigma or even a divine punishment. Those ideas became further sophisticated as the attention this issue received increased, and as infertility was discussed on different grounds.

Advice Books for Married Couples as a Site of Infertility Debate

The stress on family is fundamental to the books on infertility, which take family as the basic unit within which this problem is observed and should be cured. The family is a sacred institution, the *raison d'être* of which is to reproduce. Hence, voluntary childlessness, rejecting to have children as well as having children outside the family bond are despicable. In Ottoman society, it was indeed a rarity to choose childlessness, yet the books on infertility talk about this choice as an oddity, as if those making this choice lack something fundamental, which is the desire to reproduce and to nurture. The absence of an elaborate discussion of voluntary childlessness is partly the result of social structures that made having children an economic necessity, but it is also a sign of the lack of proper vocabulary to comprehend and express this choice. The sacred bond of family is the child according to the literature on infertility. A marriage that remains barren is believed to be a stage to a never ending debate, quarrel, and sorrow.[41] Only a marriage with children can enjoy harmony and happiness. It is for this reason, Avazade Süleyman mentions, childless couples have sought help from many different sources, including both religion and superstition. However, most of them failed to have a child despite the sacrifices offered, sacred verses read over and over, fumigations, or the money spent to the 'quacks'.[42]

As I discussed Chapter 4, the late nineteenth and early twentieth century witnessed the proliferation of advice literature. As part of this trend, many writers turned their attention to family and marriage, and wrote advice books targeting married couples, or those about to get married. Within the peculiar context of Ottoman pronatalism, as the literature on infertility stressed the importance of family bond, advice literature about marriage turned into a heated site of debate related to infertility. Prescriptive literature counselling married couples is a prolific area to discuss and reconstruct Ottoman pronatalism. Fertility, infertility, and fecundity are among the favourite topics of this genre. The marriage handbooks always discuss infertility as a source of problem even as a calamity hindering the happiness of the couples. These books also devote their pages to describing the causes and cures of infertility. Nusret Fuad's *İzdivac: Şerait-i Sıhhiye ve İctimaiyesi*, Hüseyin Remzi's *Sağdıç-Rehber-i İzdivaç* were the earlier examples of this genre. After the turn of the century especially within the political context of Second Constitutional period, such books literary flourished.

Besim Ömer's also wrote advice books for married couples. His views about fertility can also be found in his *Sıhhatnüma-yı İzdivaç* and *Fenn-i İzdivaç* besides his medical book *Ukum ve Ananet*. His admonitions for couples are situated in between medicine and advice literature. As I discussed above, in his medical book on infertility and impotence, *Ukum ve Ananet*, Besim Ömer discussed the medical and physiological causes of infertility in great detail. In *Sıhhatnüma-yı İzdivaç* he handles the causes and cures of infertility as part of a problem threatening marriages. In this work, he emphasizes the importance of cleanliness, hygiene, and healthiness of genitals to ensure fertility.[43] However, he gives more space to social and personal factors such as character, age, lifestyle, income, the climate, as well as race and heredity as having impact on fertility.

Despite the emphasis on personal and social causes of infertility, he does not retreat from the medicalization approach and does not concede to constructing infertility as a moral problem. According to him, infertility is not seen as a divine punishment as opposed to the other prescriptive books of this genre.

According to prescriptive literature on marriage, infertility is a problem that hinders the peace and happiness of the family and leaves the real target of marriage, which is to produce offspring, null. These books discuss the factors that affect fertility and that may cause infertility, in addition to proposing possible cures or solutions. The prescriptive literature positions infertility predominantly as result of a fault or wrongdoing of the couple. In other words, most of such works assert that the couple must be doing something wrong and hence calling infertility deliberately or unconsciously. The fault of the couple might be related to the timing of sexual activity, the things they eat, or the physical conditions of their bedroom. It was supposed that when these factors are corrected, the couple would be able to overcome infertility and to have children. Sometimes the age or the character of the husband and wife might be causing infertility, but even in such cases, the prescriptive literature believes, correct diet or some changes in the lifestyle would be helpful. The marriage handbooks also discuss the importance of cleanliness and hygiene as one of the major factors influencing fertility.

Nusret Fuad, for example, sees infertility mostly as a problem related to the conditions surrounding sexual intercourse, the target of which is reproduction. Hygiene, cleanliness, the concentration of the couples on the sexual activity, the nature of the relationship between them, their mood, noisiness of the room are among many such factors that affect fertility. According to him, the couples should get involved in sexual activity (*fiil-i cima*) always under pure silence and serenity (*sukut ve istirahat*). Lack of cleanliness would cause disgust and in the long run hate and coldness among the couples, and as a result it would lead to the decline in fertility. Nusret Fuad also advises husbands to pay attention to the mood of their wives. He tells the husband to make sure that his wife is not sick or unhappy, and not to force them in this case. He also mentions that husbands should avoid violence and coarseness toward their wives, and that they should behave tender and friendly. According to Nusret Fuad, the failure to follow these basic rules would lead to infertility.[44]

Nusret Fuad tells that infertility affects both men and women and it is the lack of ability to generate or the incapability to survive one's descent.[45] He notes that in the ancient times, infertility/infecundity was seen as a stigma and once it was found out that husband or wife lacks the ability to generate, he or she was legally ordered to divorce. This seems to be the best and most appropriate solution according to Nusret Fuad, who asserts that he agrees with that ancient rule, and does not approve of a marriage which would not produce any offspring.

According to him, similar to other marriage hand books, the real goal or the *reason-d'être* of marriage is to produce offspring.

Despite this moralistic standpoint condemning infertility as a punishment, he feels the necessity to tell that it is mostly physiological and medical problems such as the total absence or mal-constitution of genitals, lack of the uterus or the ovum, the deficiencies in the constitution of the uterus and cervix, or some infections are the most common causes of infertility. Nusret Fuad also stresses the addiction to masturbate (*istimnad bi-l-yed*), age, personal traits, and overweight would cause infertility.[46] He mentions that, especially for men, excessive sexual intercourse and masturbation would lead to the lack and deficiency of semen and lead to infertility if not impotence.[47] Masturbation is emphasized as one of the major reasons of infertility and impotence in the books on impotence.[48]

Avanzade Süleyman's *Mesail-i Mühimmeden Kısır Kadınlar* underlines hygiene and cleanliness as a crucial factor influencing fertility, and advocates his female readers to take good care of their genitalia. He asserts that a woman has two very important and precious organs, which are her mount and her vagina. Although both of those have to be kept pure and clean, many women fail to do that. When she has a sickness or a problem with her genitalia, her mind and body would not be free of disease, either.[49] The literature also mentions than in many cases when a woman complains about her physical or health problems, the real problem turns out to be with the genitals. Prescriptive literature, accordingly, tells elaborately how to take care of genitalia, how to wash the vagina.

Besim Ömer in his marriage handbook converges to the other advice books' conceptualization of infertility when he is talking about the importance of hygiene and cleanliness. For example, in his advice to married couples, he points out the link between the health and well constitution of the genitals and fertility. Cleanliness and cleaning the body as well as the vagina are also important, he says. Besim Ömer also attaches an important attention to hygiene in his other works as well. We should remember at this point that in his other works he had associated unlicensed local midwives with dirt and filthiness.[50] He was one of the founders of the filthy, old, ignorant midwife stereotype in the Ottoman context. In many of his works, he criticized the dirty hands and dirty equipment of the local midwives. In both *Ukum ve Ananet* and *Sıhhatnüma-yı İzdivaç* he talks about the importance and hygiene and points out the doctors as the agents of cleanliness. Cleanliness and hygiene cannot be achieved by washing the hand and the body with water merely according to him. He also refers to the doctors, and describes very elaborately the way a doctor should wash his hand and equipment.[51] Yet, despite the importance attached to hygiene, Besim Ömer also says that water and being too clean can be the enemy of fertilization and over washing the body might turn in to a hidden reason of infertility.[52]

Advice literature about marriage also discusses the appropriate frequency of sexual intercourse for married couples according to their age and state of their health. A healthy couple is advised to have sexual intercourse two to at most four times a week with a least one day apart.[53] Too frequent or too seldom sexual activity would result in infertility according to the prescriptive writers. As such, the normative literature conceptualizes infertility as the punishment for lack of discipline, extravagance, repulsiveness, and excessiveness. Infertility is mostly depicted as a moral problem, rather than a medical or physiological one. Although some people are infertile or impotent due to the deficiency of the sexual organs, many others prepare this calamity themselves for their wrong behaviours.

Another issue handled by the advice literature as a possible reason of infertility is the determination of the right timing for sexual activity and hence conception. These books advice that sexual activity carried out before sleep is more fertile than the one in the morning. Besim Ömer, too agrees with that idea, and discusses in a detailed way the right timing of sexual intercourse.[54] Avanzade Süleyman, similarly, tells that the best time is to have sex in the evening. He notes that women should avoid going to the bathroom and they should lie down until morning to ensure fertilization.[55] Besim Ömer notes that the time when the husband and wife are the healthiest, most powerful, and most rested is the most fertile time, as well.[56] The advice literature argues that if fertilization takes place when the mind is too much preoccupied with something else, the child would be weak and unhealthy.[57] The advice writers propose the couples to abstain from having sex for ten to fifteen days before menstruation, and get involved in sexual activity tree or four days after the menstruation to increase fertility.[58]

While fertility was seen as an important issue, the health and wellbeing of the child was also important. The advice literature assumes the link between the parents and the children. However, the nature and the mechanisms of this link are not yet clear. It is usually believed that when the parents are beautiful, smart, sturdy, the offspring will also bear similar characteristics. The explanation for the cases that this rule does not apply lies in the conditions under which the mother has conceived. When the couple is too tired or weak they should avoid sexual intercourse, since in the case of conception the child would probably be weak and tired.[59] For the best offspring, it is utmost important to determine the time and place of sexual intercourse. The couples should strictly avoid being involved with sexual activity when they are drunk, tired, or when too much preoccupied with another issue.[60]

Another issue prescriptive literature discusses in relation to infertility is the proper age for marriage. According to this genre, the failure to get married at the proper age would lead to infertility. The advice books mention that women, who marry too early or too late, after thirty five to forty, do generally lack the ability to give birth.[61] Those who marry too young would not be able to conceive since they are not physiologically fertile and not ready for reproduction.

But those who marry late would also remain infertile since they would lose their ability to reproduce as a result of leaving their reproductive capacities futile for a long time.[62] Luckily, however, this kind of infertility is curable easily though the provocation of sexual desire, according to the writers of this genre. Advice literature gives very detailed descriptions of provoking sexual desire and hence fertility, including massaging the body, stimulating blood circulation by applying stinging nettle, hitting, or even whipping.[63]

Besim Ömer, too, handles the age factor. He does not recommend getting married too young and say that early marriages would not produce offspring. He notes that it is very rare that such marriages would have a child, but in that case when a child is born, he/she would be weak, short, and sick, unfortunately.[64] Besim Ömer criticizes the Ottoman custom to marry girls too young, at the age of around twelve.[65] Women who marry and give birth when they are not developed enough would not only give birth to less children, but the children would be weaker as well.[66] As a doctor, he warns his readers that female physiology and psychology becomes ready for birth at the age of twenty.[67] As part of the advice to determine the proper age to get married and to have children, adolescence and adulthood are demarcated from each other. In other words, being able to give birth physically and being ready for parenthood mentally and emotionally are duly regarded as two separate things. Menstruation is an important topic for this discussion. It is emphasized that having menstruation is not a sign of being able to give birth.[68] Menstruation, function of the ovaries, the link between menstruation and conception are important topics in the medical and advice books alike. While the medical treatises explain the function of the ovaries, uterus and the physiology of reproduction on medical grounds, the advice literature benefit from this literature, and tap the medical language.

Halid Ziya, who always talks about quite exceptional examples to embolden his position and arguments, also gives such a case to demonstrate that menstruation, ovulation, and fertility are different issues. He mentions a girl who started to menstruate only eight days after she was born. The second example is that of a woman who was over forty and with seven children but had never menstruated.[69] Yet, apart from these extreme examples, he also agrees that best age for marriage is eighteen for women and twenty for men. Neither giving birth too young, nor the opposite, giving birth too late would produce fertile results he says. He even argues that old people should not be allowed to marry, since they would be spending their final vital energy, uselessly. Moreover, if they happen to have a child, Halid Ziya tells, that child would not be healthy, and even if he/she has a young body, would definitely have an old soul. Along these lines, he gives the example of a couple who were respectively ninety seven and a hundred and five when they married. Although they were exceptionally lucky to have three children, those poor children were born old, and at only fifteen they lost their teeth, their hair whitened, and their faces terribly wrinkled.[70] According to him, the majority of the marriages at improper ages would not produce fertile results, and those exceptional ones would have unhealthy offspring.

It is not only age but character as well that affect fertility, the prescriptive literature argues. An association between temperament and fertility is assumed in many books. Besim Ömer for examples tells that some temperaments are more suited to reproduction compared to others.[71] Women who are cold or extremely ambitious are generally infertile since the former are too stagnant and lack dynamism while the latter are excessive. Again, such types of infertility are curable, through the encouragement of the opposite behaviour.[72] This association can also be found in other books.

Nymphomania is described as the excessive desire to have and the inability to resist sexual intercourse. Besim Ömer sees this as a psychological situation. He notes that besides nymphomania, masturbation (*istimna bi-l-yed*) and excessive sexual intercourse would cause infertility.[73] It is highly probable, according to Besim Ömer that a woman who had conceived in the first intercourse would lose the embryo in the successive attempts. This issue offers an invaluable prism to see Besim Ömer's moral assumptions. He says that due to the harms of successive intercourse whores never conceive and become pregnant.[74]

The books on marriage usually touch upon the issue of abortion and miscarriage. Similar to the advice books on pregnancy, miscarriage is usually depicted as the outcome of the failure to follow a disciplined and appropriate lifestyle. Abortion, generally received lesser attention, and loathed. The risks abortion possess for the mother's life is underlined and women are advised to avoid abortion and give child birth. One of the accounts is interesting for openly advocating the legitimacy of abortion in cases when the mother's life is threatened by pregnancy and childbirth. But this account tells that under such conditions abortion should be operated by an expert and under medical conditions. When induced under medical conditions termination of pregnancy is not dangerous, since the contemporary medicine provided all kinds of medicaments and treatment.[75]

Finally, the approach that believes that fertility could be manipulated through diet and lifestyle changes figures most strongly in Halid Ziya's *Kanun ve Fenn-i Vilade*. Halid Ziya juxtaposes the question of curing infertility with the ways to knowing the sex of the child. According to him, overcoming infertility is closely related to determining whether the child would be a boy or a girl, since both issues are related to the sexual power (*kuvve-i cinsiye*) of the parents. The sexual power, according to Halid Ziya, is the degree femininity of women and the degree of masculinity of men. According to this conception, if the femininity of the mother dominates over the masculinity of the father, the child would be a girl, and he would be a boy in the opposite case.

Here Halid Ziya makes a distinction between sexual power (*kuvve-i cinsiyye*) and physical power (*kuvve-i cismaniye*).[76] Physical strength is different from sexual power and being physically strong and sturdy does not always assure a high sexual power. But what exactly is the nature of the sexual power? Halid Ziya tells that femininity and masculinity is encapsulated in the ovum (*madde-i beyze*), which is the cell that contains the essence of femininity or masculinity.[77] However, Halid Ziya laments that contemporary medicine cannot tell exactly the nature and mechanisms of femininity and masculinity.[78] He expects that, once the science of medicine finds out more about this issue researches to find out whether it is possible to determine the sex of the child will be carried out. However, Halid Ziya notes, the degree of the sexual power could be estimated through the observation of the face and the body. For example if a woman looks more similar to her father and grandfathers than her mother and grandmothers, we can conclude that her degree of masculinity (*tezekküriyet*) is higher than her femininity and she will most probably give birth to a son, while a woman who resembles her mother and grandmother has more femininity and would presumably give birth to a daughter.[79]

Age also affects the power of masculinity and femininity according to Halid Ziya. He tells that the power of masculinity is not strong enough before twenty and after forty five years of age, and therefore those who become fathers when their power of masculinity is low would mostly have daughters. The balance of the power of masculinity and femininity between the couples is also important. And accordingly, when, for example, the mother's power of femininity reigns over the father's power of masculinity the couple would most likely have a daughter, while they should expect a son in the opposite case.[80]

Along these lines, it is also possible to manipulate the sexual power through changing and regulating the lifestyle and diet. For example, a woman with a high degree of masculinity is most likely to be thin with small breasts and very active. To increase her femininity, she should adopt a more peaceful and silent lifestyle, and eat more to put on some more weight. She should go out less and sleep more.[81] Halid Ziya even cites a research which was alleged to be carried out with a sample of a hundred women, who changed their lifestyles and diet accordingly to make them fit to give birth to daughters. Seventy-eight of them gave birth to daughters and only twenty-two failed.[82] Having some illnesses and having weak nerves is also associated with giving birth to daughters. In order to have a son, one should first be cured.[83] If a couple wants to have a boy, the masculine power of the mother should be provoked by a protein-rich diet, having cold showers, lots of physical activity, and little sleep.[84] Such a lifestyle would eventually decrease her femininity and increase masculinity.

This discussion offers us rich insights about the assumptions about femininity and masculinity. It is also significant that the ways for increasing or decreasing femininity and masculinity is always exemplified through women. Although father's degree of masculinity is mentioned at the beginning, it is not problematized afterwards. And not the fathers but the mothers are advised to change their lifestyles, diet and physical activity.

Here Halid Ziya refers to a case as told by Auguste Debay. He talks about two families which are acquainted with each other. Their daughters and sons cross marry and one couple happens to have six daughters, other five sons, whereas the third fail to have any child at all in the meantime. The first couple loss their wish and hope to have a son and stop trying another pregnancy. The second couple believes that that many sons is enough and stop planning another child. But the couple, who lack any child, do not give up trying and happen to come across Debay's book on fertility when they were searching for a cure for their childlessness. They immediately buy the book, read it, and start to practice the admonitions expressed in it. By strictly following Debay's prescriptions, they manage to have a child a while later. Encouraged by their success, the other couples decide to try the same method, the first to have a son and the other to have a daughter respectively. The first couple manages to have a baby boy following Debay's method, whereas the latter fail to have a daughter and their newborn baby turns out to be yet another boy. The husband admits that his wife is just too masculine, and since she was not patient enough to follow the diet and changes in her lifestyle and physical activity that Debay's book recommends, she was not able to increase her femininity and decrease her masculinity. But when the other couples insisted too much, they decided to have another try, and the wife finally managed to change her diet and activity, and to increase her power of femininity. Finally, she was able give birth to a daughter thanks to her increased femininity.[85] This example by Halid Ziya is one of the strongest evidence of his belief that femininity and masculinity could be manipulated through diet and lifestyles. Halid Ziya also tells that breeding animals or plants is seen as its proof.[86]

Finally, despite the discourses on the importance of having a good number of children, some people who are more fertile and fecund than it was pleased are seen as another source of problem. The books on family stress that point especially toward the end of the century when Ottoman pronatalist policies were quite consolidated. For example, in *Fenn-ü İzdivac* Besim Ömer criticizes the idea that a woman should give birth as much as possible.[87] Mothering is a sacred duty which requires a high amount of sacrifice from the mother. But a woman who has one baby in the crib, one baby on her lap, and yet one in her belly obviously cannot do this duty adequately. Along these lines, Besim Ömer advocates the disciplining of fertility.[88] Although motherhood is the most sacred and important of all humanitarian duties, it is at the same time the most demanding and most difficult of them all. Hence it should not be exaggerated (*ifrada kaçmamalı*). Yet here Besim Ömer talks about three to five children, not less, as normal, and he even gives a chart in his book that shows the best timing to be able to give birth to five children in total.[89] In *Mesail-i Mühimme*, Avanzade

Süleyman also mentions that in Ottoman society, it is usually the poor who give birth to larger number of children, and the wealthier and affluent families tend to have smaller number of children. As a result the culture of the poor is enhanced while share of the wealthier, educated, moral population decreases gradually.[90] Moreover, the poor become poorer and poorer. Such assumptions usually end with advice to poor families to give birth to children that they can take care of. Another aspect of such debates is the advice about how to avoid pregnancy. But *Mesail-i Mühimmeden Kısır Kadınlar* tell women/men how to take precaution against conception.[91] The emergence of this debate should also be analyzed together with the changing discourses of Ottoman pronatalism. The transformation of the debate on infertility was parallel with the transformation of the debate on precautions and discipline during pregnancy. And after the turn of the century it would be possible to see more outspoken examples of those eugenic ideas. Although it is a much later example the publication of a book titled *Gebe Kalmamak İçin Ne Yapmalı*? (What to do in order to Avoid Pregnancy)[92] can be made meaningful only within this context.

Although the whole issue of Ottoman pronatalism was about fertility and the ways of increasing it, its exact opposite, infertility, was not discussed in explicit ways until the late century. The books on pregnancy hinted that infertility and childlessness was a tragedy, while the choice not to have children was seen as a signpost of debauchery. It was only towards the end of the century that Ottoman medical elites and intellectuals turned their attention directly to infertility and sought ways of curing it. The cure of infertility denied the role of local midwives who had undertaken this role for centuries. It accordingly saw the doctors as the active agents of recovering this reproductive dysfunction. The male body, largely overlooked by pronatalist policies, was also problematized by the discourses on infertility. Although the books on infertility mostly constructed women as passive patients to be cured by doctors, it is important that the burden of infertility was not thrown merely on women. Thus, the debates on male reproductive dysfunctions and impotence shows that twentieth-century pronatalism would be different than the pronatalism of the Tanzimat period analysed throughout this book. Similar to the debates on care during pregnancy, a close reading of the books on infertility also hint that pronatalism would deal more with who should reproduce and who should not in the coming century and in the early Republic, which is a crucial topic that should be investigated by future studies.

CONCLUSION: GENDERING NINETEENTH-CENTURY OTTOMAN HISTORY

In this work, I have explored the gendered ways in which the fear of depopulation was articulated in the mid to late nineteenth-century Ottoman society and discussed Ottoman pronatalism. In order to present the specificities of Ottoman pronatalism, I analysed the multiple devices through which women's bodies were subjected to medical, institutional and legal scrutiny as an integral part of the search for solutions to population loss. In my analysis of the meanings of gender in the pronatalist debates, I argued that political change, demographic transformation, the emerging notions of public health and medical developments were all overlapping processes. In this sense, this book seeks to discuss the meanings of political power, Ottoman identity and medicine through the lens of gender in late Ottoman society. In order to contextualize this broad problematic, it focuses its attention on the specific issues of the transformation of midwifery, the anti-abortion debate and the medicalization of pregnancy and childbirth, respectively.

Starting from the mid-nineteenth century, the previously female spheres of pregnancy, childbirth, abortion and infertility became topics of public debate. In this period, the fecundity of women, maternal death rates and the conditions before, during and after childbirth attracted the attention of a major portion of Ottoman statesmen and doctors. In addition, an array of new social practices accompanied and reinforced this attention. During this time in Ottoman society, a midwifery school was established to medically instruct the profession, and also to license and regulate midwives; abortion was banned by laws; poor families were given financial help to encourage them to have more children; after several failed attempts, a maternity clinic was finally opened; and the first examples of advice books, which advocate medical control during pregnancy, were published for the benefit of pregnant women. Pronatalism received increasing consideration as a component of the discussions regarding the fate of the Ottoman country.

The core of Ottoman pronatalism was woven from threads connected to the anxieties of depopulation and the new practices of state rule. Through the course of the nineteenth century, the Ottoman state was deprived of a drastic amount of population due to territorial losses, nationalist rebellions and the formation of independent states, vast migration movements and epidemics. The prevalent demographicist ideology, equating the magnitude of population with economic, international, and military power, further enhanced Ottoman anxieties about depopulation. Once it became ineffective in controlling these broader factors, the Ottoman state turned its attention to the female sphere of reproduction and searched for the possible means of increasing birth rates and decreasing maternal death rates in order to counterbalance the population decrease.

In the nineteenth century, a larger population was also the precondition of the new administrative mentality that was defined on an array of mutual rights and responsibilities. Starting with Mahmud II's rule, a process redefining the relationship between the state and subjects became prevalent. This process found its expression in the criminal code of 1840, the land reform of 1858, the new juridical foundations, changes in legislation, bans on the slave trade, the provision of education, health, infrastructure services and enhanced transportation and communication facilities that were steadily made available to larger portions of the population. The administrative, educational and infrastructural planning was dependent upon creating a large population base and having a concrete hold on its size, composition and mobility. Thus, I argue, Ottoman pronatalism was an integral component of the social and political changes in the nineteenth century.

Whatever the shortcomings or strengths of these overlapping processes, they created not only a new sense of population, but also of femininity. Throughout the course of the century, women received unprecedented attention as the bearers of the future Ottoman population. The different aspects of female reproduction – pregnancy, childbirth, abortion and infertility – came under legal, medical and institutional control. However, I have argued that this process could not be stigmatized as absolute control over female bodies, but entailed opportunities for women's agency. To make it more specific, in return for bearing the children needed for a prosperous country, women received their share in the promised redefinition of the relationship between the Ottoman state and society.

Starting with the establishment of the Midwifery School in 1842, the Ottoman state increasingly sought to license midwives and regulate their activities. Being licensed became the main marker of difference and the main source of opposition among midwives. Moreover, in this period, a medical hierarchy was established and midwives were placed at its lowest echelons. However, it would not be correct to conclude that midwives were victimized by the official regulations; they also won in this process. Although they were placed at the bottom of the medical hierarchy, they started to enjoy newly earned benefits, such as retirement, pension, sick leave and other financial aid. With the petitions they sent to the government, they sought to protect their newly earned rights.

Through a detailed examination of the official correspondence regarding these regulations, I have sought to demonstrate that the transformation of midwifery and the reconstruction of the medical enterprise was not a state project formulated at the highest offices and imposed on those below. Mainstream historiography, at one and the same time, sees the Ottoman state as either an omnipotent entity or a demising one, based on its presumed inability to cope with 'modern' ways of rule and creating wealth. A critical examination of the regulation of midwifery, however, challenges the standard ways of conceptualizing the Ottoman state. The investigation of the regulation of midwifery specifically, and the medical developments more generally, demonstrates that neither view could represent the role of the Ottoman state in the particular questions of this research. A chronological reading of the regulation of midwifery suggests that the Ottoman state was an amalgam of different local and central offices, which varyingly communicated, gave consent, opposed one another and negotiated. Furthermore, Ottoman women and men were also involved in this process by expressing their wishes and grievances through petitions, demanding educated midwives and reporting malpractice.

Another major element of Ottoman pronatalism through which Ottoman bureaucrats and medical elites sought to regulate the fecundity of women was the anti-abortion debate. In this period, a major portion of Ottoman bureaucrats and intellectuals argued that abortion was the main reason for the scarcity of the population, and hence, that it should be banned. In the initial stages of this debate, until the late 1850s, the anti-abortion stance appropriated a language that stressed morality and religion to discourage abortions. According to this discourse, abortion was the act of immoral women who avoided bearing children and raising them due to their debauchery. However, as it became clear that this discourse would not help deter abortions, a more neutral language emphasizing economic hardship was used instead. In addition, financial aid was offered to families with more than seven, and later more than four children, and to those having twins. It is also significant that in this period, the Ottoman state shunned punishing women who had abortions and instead imposed punishment on those who procured the necessary means for them.

The analysis of the anti-abortion debate also brings forward important questions regarding the agency of women in Ottoman society. Despite their differences, the different legal schools of Islam, which was the dominant frame of law for the Muslim populations of the empire until the nineteenth century, allowed abortion when the mother's life was at risk. However, the Tanzimat laws on abortion criminalized this practice unconditionally. Although this situation might be evaluated as a sign of state control over the female body, I argue that it was through these laws that Ottoman women were addressed, for the first time, directly by the Ottoman state, thereby gaining legal agency. Thus, ironically, the subjection of reproduction to state laws promised Ottoman women, for the first time, a share in the new relationship between the state and society.

The anti-abortion debate, moreover, explicitly demonstrates that the fears of depopulation were not about protecting the extant demographic composition, but were limited to the fate of the 'Muslim' population. Although the historical evidence presented here is limited at this stage, the available documentation suggests that pronatalist bureaucrats and intellectuals openly lamented that it was the Muslims whose population was declining due to the widespread occurrence of abortion, and that it was Muslims who undertook military service, whereas non-Muslims and especially the Christians of the empire enjoyed higher population growth rates thanks to the lack of these two unfavourable factors. The preoccupation of the pronatalist parties with the Muslim population highlights the shortcomings of the Tanzimat ideals and the promise of equality among Ottoman subjects regardless of faith, ethnicity and social status. In sum, a critical examination of the anti-abortion debate shows that the anxieties of depopulation embodied at least the rudiments of a process associating being 'Ottoman' with being 'Muslim' despite all the commitments made by the Tanzimat.

As the third component of the pronatalist policies, I examined the medicalization of childbirth and pregnancy. Besides medical and institutional changes, the discourses were also part and parcel of the politics of the female body. For this particular purpose, I analysed the prescriptive literature for pregnant women. The emergence of such prescriptive literature is complementary with the wider medical, legal and institutional developments elaborated on in the previous chapters. While the Ottoman government encouraged women to bear larger numbers of children, it also, for the first time, took the health and wellness of these children as important goals and this frame assumed healthy pregnancy as the landmark of healthy future generations. However, I have argued that despite its disciplinary functions, the prescriptive literature assigned an important degree of agency to Ottoman women, who, in the last analysis, were to make the best decisions for themselves and for their children.

Finally, I examined infertility as another site of Ottoman pronatalism. Although the politics of female reproduction centred on the question of fertility and fecundity, the issue of infertility and reproductive experiences about it were not directly addressed until the late century. The cases of involuntary childlessness and the reproductive dysfunctions first attracted the attention of medical doctors. The medicalization of infertility constructed this problem as an abnormality and the infertile as a patient to be cured. However, shortly non-medical works on infertility also emerged as part of the debates on population increase, and normative and popular works welcomed this issue as an opportunity to express broader concerns about the anxieties of demography. Besides offering clues about the conceptualization of femininity, the debates on infertility also problematize the male body. As such, books on infertility are a rare field where Ottoman pronatalism targeted the male body and reproductive experience beside the female ones. Moreover, along with the pregnancy handbooks, the documents on infertility hint the early premises of eugenic ideas as conceived by the Ottoman doctors and intellectuals.

Although the scholarship in Ottoman history is becoming increasingly sophisticated, it is for the most part written in terms of institutional and legal transformations, which, unfortunately, remained ignorant of women and gender. In this work, I have tried to reinterpret the renowned stories of the long nineteenth century from a gendered perspective. To do that, I used gender both as a method of historical analysis and as a topic of historical research. Empirically, I tried to unearth women's experiences of reproduction women in Ottoman society. Methodologically, I used gender as a tool of historical analysis to discuss the changing meanings of femininity and the different situations of power in Ottoman society.

At the heart of this book is the argument that in the late Ottoman history, pregnancy, childbirth and abortion were not personal experiences but political subjects. In this sense, investigation of Ottoman pronatalism challenges and reshapes the standard dichotomy between 'public' and 'private' by blurring the boundaries between the 'political' and the 'personal', 'state' and 'family'. As such, looking through the lens of gender offers a new and fresh reinterpretation of the long nineteenth century. To conclude, the analysis of the ways in which gender permeated the definition of the state and society relationship will contribute to the complex history this book has only started to tackle – that of the relationship between the intimate and the political.

NOTES

For abbreviations to archive material and title translations, please see the Works Cited.

Introduction

1. For discussions of 'Ottomanism' see Ş. Hanioğlu, 'Osmanlıcılık', in *Tanzimattan Cumhuriyete Türkiye Ansiklopedisi*, 5 (İstanbul: İletişim Yayınevi, 1985), pp. 1389–93; Ş. Mardin, *The Genesis of Young Ottoman Thought: A Study in the Modernization of Turkish Political Ideas* (Syracuse, NY: Syracuse University Press, 2000). For a much recent work, see S. A. Somel, 'Osmanlı Reform Çağında Osmanlıcılık Düşüncesi (1839–1913)', in M. Belge (ed.), *Modern Türkiye'de Siyasi Düşünce: Tanzimat ve Cumhuriyet'in Birikimi* (Istanbul: İletişim Yayınevi, 2001), pp. 88–116.
2. For discussions of public sphere in the Ottoman context, see E. Frierson, 'Unimagined Communities: Women and Education in the Late-Ottoman Empire, 1876–1909', *Critical Matrix, The Princeton Journal of Women, Gender, and Culture*, 9:2 (1995), pp. 55–90; C. Kırlı, 'The Struggle Over Space: Coffeehouses of Ottoman Istanbul 1780–1845' (PhD dissertation, Binghamton University, 2000); C. Kırlı, 'Coffeehouses: Public Opinion in the Nineteenth Century Ottoman Empire', in A. Salvatore and D. F. Eickelman (eds), *Public Islam and the Common Good* (Brill Academic Publishers, 2004), pp. 75–97; C. Kırlı, 'Kahvehaneler ve Hafiyeler: 19. Yüzyıl Ortalarında Osmanlı'da Sosyal Kontrol', *Toplum ve Bilim*, 83 (2000), pp. 58–79; N. Özbek, *Osmanlı İmparatorluğu'nda Sosyal Devlet, Siyaset, İktidar ve Meşruiyet, 1876–1914* (Istanbul: İletişim Yayınevi, 2002); N. Özbek, 'Defining the Public Sphere during the Late Ottoman Empire: War, Mass Mobilization and the Young Turk Regime (1908–18)', *Middle Eastern Studies*, 43:5 (2007), pp. 795–809. See also N. Turna, 'Pandemonium and Order: Suretyship, Surveillance, and Taxation in Early Nineteenth Century Istanbul', *New Perspectives on Turkey*, 39 (2008), pp. 167–89; E. E. Akşit, 'Geç Osmanlı ve Cumhuriyet Dönemlerinde Nüfus Kontrolü Yaklaşımları', *Toplum ve Bilim*, 118 (2010), pp. 179–97; F. Özbay, 'Türkiye'de ulus-devlet, gözetim ve nüfus bilgisi', *Toplum ve Bilim*, 118 (2010), pp. 165–78.
3. Despite increasingly sophisticated work on population and demography, we still do not have reliable data about the growth rate of the Ottoman population in the nineteenth century. One main problem is the lack of information about the diverse growth rates between the different religious/ethnic groups. Due to the nature of the sources available, pinning down accurate estimates of fertility rates is an almost impossible task, yet this excuse is over-exploited in the works which remain bluntly ignorant about the diversities between different groups along the lines of ethnicity, religion and class. For a discussion

on fertility rates, see C. Behar and A. Duben, *Istanbul Households: Marriage, Family and Fertility, 1880–1940* (New York: Cambridge University Press, 2002), especially chapter 6, 'Fertility and Birth Control: Istanbul's Particularities', pp. 159–93. Moreover, assessing the fertility rates which is pivotal to this kind of a research is also a difficult task. One of the most comprehensive studies on Ottoman population, K. Karpat's work also acknowledges the problems of studying the population in Ottoman history as well as some of the problems of the historiography. He also reminds of the caveat of ignoring the differences in growth rates between Muslim and non-Muslim groups. Karpat notes that it is generally assumed that during the first thirty years of the nineteenth century the Ottoman population decreased, beginning to increase again after 1850. The non-Muslim population actually grew at a fairly fast rate after the 1830s – probably 2 per cent annually; the Muslim population declined or remained the same in number. There are indications, however, that fertility rates among the Muslims began to increase after 1850. See K. Karpat, *Ottoman Population, 1830–1914* (Madison, WI: University of Wisconsin Press, 1985).

4. D. Quataert, 'The Age of Reforms, 1812–1914', in H. İnalcık and D. Quataert (eds), *An Economic and Social History of the Ottoman Empire* (New York: Cambridge University Press, 1997), pp. 759–943, on p. 777.
5. D. Quataert, *The Ottoman Empire: 1700–1922* (New York: Cambridge University Press, 2000), p. 112.
6. Karpat, *Ottoman Population*, pp. 160–1. K. Karpat, 'Ottoman Population Records and the Census of 1881/82–1893', *International Journal of Middle East Studies*, 9:3 (1978), pp. 237–74, on p. 246.
7. Karpat, 'Ottoman Population Records', p. 246. For a detailed account of impact of migration movements on Ottoman population, see chapter 4, 'Population Movements in the Ottoman State in the Nineteenth Century', in Karpat, *Ottoman Population*, pp. 60–85.
8. The 1857 İskan Kararnamesi declared that migration into the Ottoman state was open to anyone who was willing to give his allegiance to the sultan, to become his subject and to respect the country's laws. The benefits of settling down in Ottoman lands were high: the immigrants would be protected against any infringement of their religious observances and enjoyed complete religious freedom. Accordingly if the place they settled did not have any chapels or churches where they could conduct their rites, they were promised imperial permission to build their chapels. Moreover, the government promised to give them the best arable lands for free and to exempt them from all taxes and military service for six years if they settled in Rumeli and for twelve years if they settled in Asia. On this issue, see Karpat, *Ottoman Population*, p. 62. Karpat's approach has recently been criticized by Fuat Dündar. As opposed to the conventional scholarship, Dündar argues that migration to Ottoman lands was not merely the outcome of Russian policies, but that the Ottoman state also vigorously promoted it. See F. Dündar, *Modern Türkiye'nin Şifresi: İttihat ve Terakki'nin Etnisite Mühendisliği (1913–1918)* (Istanbul: İletişim Yayınevi, 2008).
9. For discussions on the populationist approaches in other national contexts, see S. Szreter, *Fertility, Class and Gender in Britain, 1860–1940* (New York: Cambridge University Press, 1996); S. Patriarca, *Numbers and Nationhood: Writing Statistics in Nineteenth-Century Italy* (New York: Cambridge University Press, 1996); A. Davin, 'Imperialism and Motherhood', in F. Cooper and A. L. Stoler (eds), *Tensions of Empire: Colonial Cultures in a Bourgeois World* (Berkeley, CA: University of California Press, 1997), pp. 87–151; J. H. Cole, *The Power of Large Numbers: Population, Politics, and Gender in*

Nineteenth-Century France (Ithaca, NY: Cornell University Press, 2000); E. Camiscioli, 'Producing Citizens, Reproducing the "French Race": Immigration, Demography, and Pronatalism in Early Twentieth-Century France', *Gender & History*, 13:3 (2001), pp. 593–621.

10. S. Dursun, 'Population Policies of the Ottoman State in the Tanzimat Era: 1840–1870' (MA Thesis, Sabancı University, 2001).
11. Karpat, *Ottoman Population*, pp. 61–2.
12. D. Quataert, *Ottoman Manufacturing in the Age of Industrial Revolution* (New York: Cambridge University Press, 1993); Quataert, 'The Age of Reforms'; Ş. Pamuk, *The Ottoman Empire and European Capitalism, 1820–1913* (New York: Cambridge University Press, 1987); M. Palairet, *The Balkan Economies, c. 1800–1914. Evolution without Development* (New York: Cambridge University Press, 1997).
13. The works on this issue are too numerous and too well-known to cite. However, for the changing bureaucracy and formation of government offices in the context of the Tanzimat reforms, see C. V. Findley, *Bureaucratic Reform in the Ottoman Empire: The Sublime Porte, 1789–1922* (Princeton, NJ: Princeton University Press, 1980); A. Akyıldız, *Tanzimat Dönemi Osmanlı Merkez Teşkilatında Reform* (Istanbul: Eren, 1993); A. Akyıldız, *Osmanlı Bürokrasisi ve Modernleşme* (Istanbul: İletişim Yayınevi, 2004). For the centralization and changing functions of the state, see K. Karpat, 'The Transformation of the Ottoman State, 1789–1908', *International Journal of Middle East Studies*, 3:3 (1972), pp. 243–81; İ. Ortaylı, *İmparatorluğun En Uzun Yüzyılı* (Istanbul: Hil Yayınevi, 1983).
14. Ariel Salzmann calls this new notion of subjectivity 'protocitizenship'. Although I will not discuss this issue in detail here, her perspective and arguments are also thought-provoking for this research. Whereas I tried to limit my perspective to the increasing attention given to population with fiscal, military and economic exigencies, the transformations in economy, politics and society were resiliently interrelated with a changing conception of subjectivity. For this reason it was not a coincidence that security of life, honour and property of the Ottoman people were secured in tandem with each other. See A. Salzmann, 'Citizens in Search of a State: The Limits of Political Participation in the Late Ottoman Empire', in M. Hanagan and C. Tilly, *Extending Citizenship, Reconfiguring States* (New York: Rowman and Littlefield Publishers, 1999), pp. 37–66.
15. For a detailed discussion of the *malikane* system, see A. Salzmann, 'Measures of Empire: Tax Farming and the Ottoman Ancien Regime,1695–1807' (PhD dissertation, Columbia University, 1995); E. Özvar, *Osmanlı Maliyesinde Malikane Uygulaması* (Istanbul: Kitabevi, 2003); Ş. Pamuk, *The Ottoman Empire*; Ş. Pamuk, *Osmanlı-Türkiye İktisadi Tarihi, 1500–1914* (Istanbul: İletişim Yayınevi, 2005). For the centralization and changing functions of the state, see Karpat, 'The Transformation of the Ottoman State,' p. 81; and Ortaylı, *İmparatorluğun En Uzun Yüzyılı*.
16. E. Z. Karal, *Osmanlı Tarihi, 1. Cilt Nizam-ı Cedid ve Tanzimat Devirleri (1789–1856)* (Türk Tarih Kurumu, 1988), pp. 263–4.
17. For the legal and institutional transformation of Ottoman taxation structures during the Tanzimat era, as well as the list of the newly introduced taxes and the other means of revenue see S. J. Shaw, 'The Nineteenth-Century Ottoman Tax Reforms and Revenue System', *International Journal of Middle East Studies*, 6:4 (1975), pp. 421–59; C. Çakır, *Tanzimat Dönemi Osmanlı Maliyesi* (Istanbul: Küre Yayınları, 2001); A. Şener, *Tanzimat Dönemi Osmanlı Vergi Sistemi* (Istanbul: İşaret Yayınları, 1990). For the share of taxes in the Ottoman budget, see M. Genç and E. Özvar (eds), *Osmanlı Maliyesi Kurumlar ve Bütçeler* (Istanbul: Osmanlı Bankası Arşiv ve Araştırma Merkezi, 2006).

For more conceptual approaches, see C. Kırlı, 'Yolsuzluğun İcadı: 1840 Ceza Kanunu, İktidar ve Bürokrasi', *Tarih ve Toplum Yeni Yaklaşımlar*, 4 (2006), pp. 45–119, and A. Y. Kaya, 'Vergilendirmenin Ekonomi Politiği: 19. Yüzyıl Ortasında İzmir Kadastrosu', in *İzmir'in Dünden Bugüne Sosyal ve Ekonomik GelişimiKonferansı Bildirileri* (İzmir: İzmir Ekonomi Üniversitesi, İzmir İktisat Kongresi Araştırma Merkezi, 2007), pp. 67–75.

18. Although it is not the main problem facing this research, it is important to note that these changes did not arrive without social conflicts. Today there is a substantial literature discussing the links between the changed taxation practices and local uprisings. The pathbreaking research on this topic belongs to Halil İnalcık, and many of the studies investigating and discussing the application of the Tanzimat in order to understand its reception at different localities, departed from a similar problem and in part replicated his perspective by focusing mainly on the local uprisings that expressed grievances about the changes in taxation practice. See H. İnalcık, 'Application of the Tanzimat and its Social Effects', *Archivum Ottomanicum*, 5 (1973), pp. 97–128. For a recent example of this approach, see H. İnalcık and M. Seyitdanlıoğlu (eds), *Tanzimat: Değişim Sürecinde Osmanlı İmparatorluğu* (Istanbul: Phoenix, 2006). The articles in this volume deal, for the most part, with the application of the Tanzimat in different places of the empire and the majority of the articles are framed in a very similar way. A search through the thesis and dissertation database of the Higher Education Council (Yüksek Öğrenim Kurumu) also yields numerous dissertations with the title 'Application of the Tanzimat and its Social Effects in ...', which is an indication of the continuing legacy and prevalence of İnalcık's perspective. These studies are beneficial for demonstrating the grievances brought about by the changes in taxation practices.
19. The latest handbook produced by the Prime Ministry Archive states that there are 1.100 *tahrir* registers in the Prime Ministry Archive in Istanbul and 2.322 registers in the Land Registry Directorate in Ankara, covering the years between 1300 and 1882. See N. Aktaş et al., *Başbakanlık Osmanlı Arşivi Rehberi* (Istanbul: Başbakanlık Devlet Arşivleri Genel Müdürlüğü Osmanlı Arşivi Daire Başkanlığı, 2000), p. 97. The Ottoman state's neat effort to count its resources and its relatively accurate documentation also fed scholarly interest on these sources.
20. For the transformation of the Ottoman State in the nineteenth century, see Karpat, 'The Transformation of the Ottoman State'.
21. Karpat, *Ottoman Population*, pp. 6–9.
22. For a theoretical discussion on the modern censuses, see B. Anderson, *Imagined Communities: Reflections on the Origin and Spread of Nationalism* (London: Verso, 1991). For specific Ottoman cases, see B. Doumani, 'The Political Economy of Population Counts in Ottoman Palestine: Nablus, circa 1850', *International Journal of Middle East Studies*, 26:1 (1994), pp. 1–17; İ. K. Yosmaoğlu, 'Counting Bodies, Shaping Souls: The 1903 Census and National Identity in Ottoman Macedonia', *International Journal of Middle East Studies*, 38 (2006), pp. 55–77; for a case from Egypt, see K. M. Cuno and M. J. Reimer, 'The Census Registers of Nineteenth-Century Egypt: A New Source for Social Historians', *British Journal of Middle Eastern Studies*, 24:2 (1997), pp. 193–216.
23. E. Z. Karal, *Osmanlı İmparatorluğu'nda İlk Nüfus Sayımı 1831* (Ankara: Başvekalet İstatistik Umum Müdürlüğü, 1943); M. Aydın, 'Sultan II. Mahmud Döneminde Yapılan Nüfus Tahrirleri', in *Sultan II. Mahmud ve Reformları Semineri: 28–30 Haziran 1989* (Istanbul: İstanbul Üniversitesi Edebiyat Fakültesi Tarih Araştırmaları Enstitüsü, 1990), pp. 81–106. Although it is commonplace to note that the census in 1831 was the 'first' modern Ottoman census, Karpat duly criticizes this statement. He argues that the collection of taxes could not have been carried out without population data of some sort. He

also critically evaluates the first hand correspondence exchanged during the preparations for the census and demonstrates the existence of a quite sound system of population registry. Karpat, *Ottoman Population*, pp. 6–9.

24. Karpat also emphasizes this point and identifies the signing of the Paris Treaty in 1856 as a turning point in the change of population philosophy. Karpat, *Ottoman Population*, pp. 6–9.
25. M. Çadırcı, 'Tanzimat Döneminde Çıkarılan Men'i Mürur ve Pasaport Nizamnameleri', *Belgeler*, 15:19 (1993), pp. 169–81.
26. Karpat, *Ottoman Population*, p. 218.
27. Karpat, 'Ottoman Population Records', p. 246.
28. BOA C.DH 209/10410 (16.R.1253/20 July 1837).
29. BOA C.DH 270/13489 (29.Z.1257/11 January 1842).
30. For example, see BOA İ.MVL 149/4213 (08.L.1265/27 August 1849) and BOA A.MKT.UM 7/91 (25.Ra.1266/08 February 1850). In the Prime Ministry Archives, it is possible to find population registers (*Vukuat Defteri*) for many places despite the gaps in time and geographic areas. The very existence of these registers, and the way they were archived is important, and demonstrates concretely the new attention given to population count.
31. N. Keddie and B. Baron (eds), *Women in Middle Eastern History: Shifting Boundaries in Sex and Gender* (New Haven, CT: Yale University Press, 1991); M. Zilfi, *Women in the Ottoman Empire: Middle Eastern Women in the Early Modern Era* (Leiden: Brill, 1997); L. Abu-Lughod, *Remaking Women: Feminism and Modernity in the Middle East* (Princeton, NJ: Princeton University Press, 1998), and J. E. Tucker and M. Meriwether (eds), *Social History of Women and Gender in the Modern Middle East* (Boulder, CO: Westview Press, 1999).
32. D. Ze'evi, *Producing Desire: Changing Sexual Discourse in the Ottoman Middle East, 1500–1900* (Berkeley, CA: University of California Press, 2006). M. Özbek, 'The Regulation of Prostitution in Beyoglu (1875–1915)', *Middle Eastern Studies*, 46:4 (January 2010), pp. 555–68.
33. L. Peirce, *Morality Tales: Law and Gender in the Ottoman Court of Aintab* (Berkeley, CA: University of California Press, 2003); I. Agmon, *Family & Court: Legal Culture and Modernity in Late Ottoman Palestine* (Syracuse, NY: Syracuse University Press, 2006). E. Semerdjian, '*Off the Straight Path: Illicit Sex, Law, and Community in Ottoman Aleppo*' (Syracuse, NY: Syracuse University Press, 2008); see also F. Zarinebaf-Shahr, *Crime and Punishment in Istanbul, 1700–1800* (Berkeley, CA: University of California Press, 2010).
34. B. Doumani (ed.), *Family History in the Middle East: Household, Property, and Gender* (Albany, NY: University of New York Press, 2003); A. A. Sonbol (ed.), *Women, the Family, and Divorce laws in Islamic History* (Syracuse, NY: Syracuse University Press, 1996).
35. E. Frierson, 'Women in Ottoman Intellectual History', in E. Özdalga (ed.), *Late Ottoman Society: The Intellectual Heritage* (Curzon, 2005), pp. 135–62; S. A. Somel, 'Sources on the Education of Ottoman Women in the Prime Ministerial Ottoman Archive for the Period of Reforms in the Nineteenth and Early Twentieth Centuries', in A. A. Sonbol (ed.), *Beyond The Exotic: Women's Histories In Islamic Societies* (Syracuse, NY: Syracuse University Press, 2005), pp. 295–306.
36. F. Zarinebaf-Shahr, 'Women, Patronage and Charity in Ottoman İstanbul', in Sonbol, *Beyond the Exotic: Women's Histories in Islamic Societies* (Syracuse, NY: Syracuse University Press, 2005), pp. 89–101.

37. B. Tuğ, 'Politics of Honor: The Institutional and Social Frontiers of "Illicit" Sex in Mid-Eighteenth-Century Ottoman Anatolia' (PhD dissertation, New York University, 2009); E. Aykut Türker, 'Alternative Claims on Justice and Law: Rural Arson and Poison Murder in the 19th Century Ottoman Empire' (PhD dissertation, Boğaziçi University, 2011).
38. S. Delice, 'Friendship, Sociability, and Masculinity in the Ottoman Empire: An Essay Confronting the Ghosts of Historicism', *New Perspectives on Turkey*, 42 (Spring 2010), pp 103–25; M. Baer, 'Manliness, Male Virtue and History Writing at the Seventeenth-Century Ottoman Court', *Gender & History*, 20:1 (2008), pp. 128–14.
39. I. Agmon, 'Women, Class, and Gender: Muslim Jaffa and Haifa at the Turn of the 20th Century', *International Journal of Middle East Studies*, 30:4 (1998), pp. 477–500; M. Baer, 'Islamic Conversion Narratives of Women: Social Change and Gendered Religious Hierarchy in Early Modern Ottoman İstanbul', *Gender & History*, 16:2 (2004), pp. 425–58; D. Ze'evi, 'Women in 17th-Century Jerusalem: Western and Indigenous Perspectives', *International Journal of Middle East Studies*, 27:2 (1995), pp. 157–73; A. Buturovic and I. C. Schick (eds), *Women in the Ottoman Balkans: Gender, Culture and History* (London: I. B. Tauris, 2007).
40. Although the place, role and limitations of court records for writing the history of women and gender in the Ottoman Empire has been quite elaborately debated, similar discussion for official documents wait to be done. See D. Ze'evi, 'The Use of Ottoman *Sharia* Court Records as a Source for Middle Eastern Social History: A Reappraisal', *Islamic Law and Society*, 5:1 (1998), pp. 35–56, and I. Agmon, 'Women, Class, and Gender'. pp. 477–500.

1 Besim Ömer and Writing the History of Midwifery and Childbirth

1. For Besim Ömer's eugenicist ideas, see B. Ömer, *'Türk Çocuğunu Nasıl Yaşatmalı?'* (Istanbul: Ahmed Ihsan Basımevi, 1939).
2. This brief biography of Besim Ömer is based mainly on the Besim Ömer Akalın file in the library of the History of Medicine and Deontology Department of Cerrahpaşa Faculty of Medicine, Istanbul.
3. For an excellent criticism of this approach in the wider scholarship of Ottoman history, see R. A. Abou-El-Haj, *Formation of the Modern State: The Ottoman Empire, Sixteenth to Eighteenth Centuries* (Syracuse, NY: Syracuse University Press, 2005).
4. Besim Ömer, *Doğum Tarihi* (Istanbul: Ahmet İhsan Matbaası, 1932).
5. I will handle the use of forceps, its role in the transformation of the knowledge of childbirth as well as the historiographical approaches regarding this role in Chapter 2.
6. Again, I will discuss in more detail the criticism of this paradigm to which Besim Ömer subscribed like many other obstetrician historians in the next chapter. However, for one of the criticisms on this issue, see M. Lindemann, 'Professionals? Sisters? Rivals? Midwives in Braunschweig, 1750–1800', in H. Marland (ed.), *The Art of Midwifery: Early Modern Midwives in Europe* (London: Routledge, 1994).
7. For a criticism of a wider criticism of internalist approaches to the history of medicine, see M. Lindemann, *Medicine and Society in Early Modern Europe* (Cambridge: Cambridge University Press, 1999), p. 2.
8. Besim Ömer, *Doğum Tarihi*.
9. Besim Ömer, 'Ebelik ve Doğum: Bizde Nasıldı ve Ne Haldedir?', in M. Osman (ed.), *Sıhhat Almanağı* (Istanbul: Kader Matbaası, 1933).

10. I will discuss the opening of the School of Midwifery and the changes in the practices of midwifery in the next chapter.
11. Besim Ömer, 'Ebelik ve Doğum?'
12. Ibid.
13. The historiography repeats that the first maternity clinic fell into disrepute as a bastard house. See, for example, F. Davis, *The Ottoman Lady: A Social History from 1718 to 1918* (Westport, CT: Greenwood Press, 1986).
14. Y. I. Ülman, 'Besim Ömer Akalın (1820–1940): Ange Gardien des Femmes et des Enfants', in M. Anastasiadou-Dumont (ed.), *Medecins et Ingenieurs Ottomans a l'age des Nationalismes* (Paris: Maisonneuve et Larose; Institut Français d'Etudes Anatoliennes, 2003); Y. I. Ülman, 'Osmanlıdan Cumhuriyete Geçiş Sürecinde Bir Aydın Portresi: Besim Ömer Akalın', *Müteferrika* 25 (2004), pp. 51–87.
15. This point has been handled by numerous works. Some of the few that can be referred to in the first place include: Ş. Hanioğlu, *The Young Turks in Opposition* (New York: Oxford University Press, 1995); Ş. Hanioğlu, *Preparation for a Revolution: The Young Turks, 1902–1908* (New York: Oxford University Press, 2001); F. Ahmad, *The Young Turks; The Committee of Union and Progress in Turkish Politics* (Oxford: Clarendon Press, 1969).
16. Besim Ömer, *Ebe Hanımlara Öğütlerim* (Istanbul: Ahmet İhsan Matbaası, 1322 (1904–5)). Besides this advice manual, Besim Ömer has also written medical treatises and guidebooks for midwives. See his translation from P. Budin, *Seririyyat-ı viladiyye dersleri*, trans. Besim Ömer (Istanbul: Mekteb-i Tıbbiyye-i Şahane Matbaası, 1313 (1895–6)); Besim Ömer, *Fenn-i Vilade*, 4 vols (Istanbul: Ahmet İhsan Matbaası, 1338 (1919–20)); and his book for midwives, Besim Ömer, *Doğurma ve Doğurtma* (Istanbul: Matbaa-i Ahmed İhsan, 1322 (1904/5)).
17. Besim Ömer, *Ebe Hanımlara Öğütlerim.*
18. Ibid.
19. Ibid.
20. Ibid. The new tasks expected from the midwives were also discussed and delineated in detail by the prescriptive literature written for pregnant women. For a more detailed discussion and analysis of this transformation and the medicalization of pregnancy and midwifery practice, see Chapter 4 of this book.
21. Ömer, *Ebe Hanımlara Öğütlerim.*
22. Ibid.
23. I will discuss these points more elaborately in Chapter 2, where I will present the regulation of midwifery in this period.
24. Ömer, *Ebe Hanımlara Öğütlerim.*
25. For its criticism, see H. Berktay, *Cumhuriyet İdeolojisi ve Fuat Köprülü* (Istanbul: Kaynak Yayınları, 1983). B. Ersanlı, *İktidar ve Tarih: Türkiye'de "Resmi Tarih" Tezinin Oluşumu (1929–1937)* (Istanbul: İletişim Yayınevi, 2003).
26. R. M. Keskin and S. Sağlık, 'Türkiyede Viladiye ve Nisaiye Tarihinden bir Hulasa', *Türk Tıp Tarihi Arkivi* (1939), pp. 101–6. For both biographies, see F. Erden, *Türk Hekimleri Biyografisi* (Istanbul: Cituri Biraderler Basımevi, 1948).
27. Most of the work on the history of medicine treats Ottoman medicine as a part of, and a natural extension to pre-Ottoman Islamic medicine. This approach not only denies credit to local medical practices and the appropriation of different medical traditions, but forges continuity throughout six centuries. The typical scheme organizes the historical narrative on a century-based periodization beginning from the

thirteenth and ending in the twentieth century, recounting the main institutions, chief physicians and the manuscripts written in each century. The result is a very synthetic, linear and monolithic account which does not address the context of any single individual event or person, or the interests unfolded in the manuscripts of physicians.

Besides these conceptual problems, the scholarship suffers some institutional problems, too. First of all, most of the historiography has been produced by doctors interested in history rather than historians. The departments of the history of medicine are not institutionalized as part of history departments but are appendages to the faculties of medicine. The two main disciplinary journals (*Tıp Tarihi Araştırmaları* and *Yeni Tıp Tarihi Araştırmaları*) are published by the two major faculties of medicine. Although being a doctor or a physician does not necessarily preclude being a good historian, and on the contrary, competence in the scientific aspects of medicine is a great skill that many historians lack; in the case of the work on Ottoman medicine, the medical background of the researchers led to an ignorance of the social aspects and meanings of medicine. Some important topics that will enlighten our understanding of the social meaning of medicine, such as diseases and epidemics, public health, madness or the commoditization of health care, are not touched on at all. Unfortunately, the problem of ignorance surrounding the social aspects of medicine is enhanced by the lack of due attention to the scientific medical questions, exactly where the works done by doctors might become a major contribution. Finally, some of the major work was published by drug companies, rather than academic publishers, which seems to be an obstacle to discussing the political issues wrapped around the medical debates.

For some of the works that are marked by this approach, see E. Kahya and A. D. Erdemir, *Medicine in the Ottoman Empire (and Other Scientific Developments)* (Nobel Tıp Kitabevleri, 1997); E. Kahya and A. D. Erdemir, *Bilimin Işığında Osmanlıdan Cumhuriyete Tıp ve Sağlık Kurumları* (Türkiye Diyanet Vakfı Yayınları, Ankara, 2000); E. Kahya and A. D. Erdemir, *Science of Medicine in the Ottoman Empire* (Hamdar Foundation, Pakistan, 2003); E. Kahya and A. D. Erdemir, *Medical Studies and Institutions in the Ottoman Empire: With Brief Information about the Scientific Studies* (Ankara: Nobel Yayın Dağıtım Tic. Ltd. Şti., 2008); E. K. Unat and M. Samasti, *Mekteb-i Tıbbiye-i Mülkiye (Sivil Tıp Mektebi) 1867–1909* (Istanbul, 1990); O. Ş. Uludağ, *Beşbuçuk Asırlık Türk Tababeti Tarihi* (Ankara: Kültür Bakanlığı, 1991); T. Riza, *Tıp Fakültesi Tarihçesi: Mir'at-ı Mektebi Tıbbiye*, ed. A. Kazancıgil (Istanbul: Özel Yayınlar, 1991); C. Yılmaz, and N. Yılmaz (eds), *Osmanlılarda Sağlık* (Istanbul: Biofarma İlaç Sanayi ve Ticaret A.Ş., 2006), B. Ak and A. Ataç (eds), *Osmanlı Devleti'nde Sağlık Hizmetleri Sempozyumu* (Ankara: Sağlık Bakanlığı, 2000).

28. For a critical appraisal of this issue, see M. S. Mossensohn, 'Tale of Two Discourses: The Historiography of Ottoman-Muslim Medicine', *Social History of Medicine*, 21:1 (2008), pp. 1–12. See also, M. S. Mossensohn, 'Health as a Social Agent in Ottoman Patronage and Authority', *New Perspectives on Turkey*, 37 (2007), pp. 147–75.
29. See, for example, B. Şehsuvaroğlu, 'Doğumun Tarihçesine ve Bizde Ebelik Öğretimine bir Bakış', *Türk Jinekoloji ve Obstetrik Mecmuası*, 4 (1967), pp. 3–4; R. Dirican, 'Türkiye'de Ebeliğin Kısa Tarihçesi', *Dirim*, 1–2 (1973).
30. B. Üstünel and E. Bayırlı, 'Ebelik ve Tarihi Gelişimi', *Zeynep Kamil Tıp Bülteni*, 3:2 (1971), pp. 67–74; Üstünel and Bayırlı, 'Ebelik ve Tarihi Gelişimi', pp. 209–16; Üstünel and Bayırlı, 'Ebelik ve Tarihi Gelişimi', pp. 1–6.
31. N. Taşkıran, 'Türkiye'de Ebelik Eğitimi', *Haseki Tıp Bülteni*, 2:3 (1973), pp. 229–40.

32. A. Kazancıgil, 'Doğum ve Kadın Hastalıkları Bilgisi', in E. K. Unat (ed.), *Tıp Dallarındaki İlerlemelerin Tarihi: Dünyada ve Türkiye'de 1850 Yılından Sonra* (Istanbul: Cerrah PaşaTıp Fakültesi Vakfı, 1988); A. Altıntaş, 'Türkiye'de Ebelik Eğitimi', in H. Hatemi and A. Altıntaş (eds), *Türk Tıp Eğitiminin Önemli Adımları* (Istanbul: CSA Global Publishing, 2006), pp. 156–60: A. H. Köker (ed.), *Doğum ve Ebelik Tarihi Kongresi, 14 Mart, 1997* (Kayseri: Kayseri Erciyes Üniversitesi Gevher Nesibi Tıp Tarihi Enstitüsü, 1997).
33. Kazancıgil, 'Doğum ve Kadın Hastalıkları Bilgisi'. His father Tevfik Remzi Kazancıgil was also one of the second generation obstetricians in the Ottoman Empire. See also the autobiographic interview book, F. Şakacı, *Her DoğumBir Mucizedir, Aykut Kazancıgil Kitabı* (Istanbul: İş Kültür Yayınları, 2005).
34. A. Süheyl, *Besim Ömer Paşa ve Doğum Tarihi* (Istanbul: Ahmet İhsan Matbaası, 1932); A. A. Onur, 'Büyük Alim ve Tıp Kahramanı, Besim Ömer Akalın', *Türk Jinekoloji Arşivi*, 24–5 (1940), pp. 1177–80; Erden, *Türk Hekimleri*, pp. 258–9; K. T. Sezenel, 'Prof. General Besim Ömer Akalın'ın Ölümü', *Türk Jinekoloji Arsivi*, 24–5 (1940), pp. 1174–6; A. M. Özden, *Doktor Besim Ömer Akalın* (Istanbul: Ahmet İhsan Matbaası, 1941); N. R. Belger, 'Türk Kadınının ve Çocuğunun Minnettar Olduğu Büyük Adam', *Akşam* (19 March 1945).
35. A. Kazancıgil, 'Ölümünün 40. Yılında Besim Ömer Paşa (1863–1940)', *Dirim*, 55 (1980), pp. 9–10; A. Akkan, 'Dr. Besim Ömer Paşa (Akalın)', *Mimar Sinan*, 6 (1992), pp. 15–20. İ. Hot, 'Besim Ömer Akalın (1862–1940)', *Yeni Tıp Tarihi Araştırmaları*, 2–3 (1996–7), pp. 213–32; Ülman, 'Besim Ömer Akalın'; Ülman, 'Osmanlıdan Cumhuriyete Geçiş'. Hot, 'Besim Ömer Paşanın Anne ve Çocuk Sağlığı Açısından Ülkemiz Nüfus Meselesi Hakkındaki Görüşleri' (MA thesis, Istanbul University, 1996), for biographic information, see especially pp. 5–26.
36. Kabile Rasiha, 'Yirmi Senelik Ebelik Hayatımda Neler Gördüm?', *Resimli Ay*, 29:21 (October 1925), pp. 43–6.
37. '50 Yıllık Ebe Sahin Anlatiyor!', *Yeni İnci*, 11:32 (1953), pp. 10–12, 16.

2 The Transformation of Midwifery

1. Biga was a town at the upper north coast of the Aegean Sea, close to Çanakkale.
2. BOA A.MKT.UM 127/96 (1269.Ca.26/10 March 1853).
3. For example, BOA İ.DH 596/41522 (1286.Ca.2/10 August 1869), BOA DH.MKT 1976/38 (1309.Z.27/23 July 1892), BOA DH.MKT 1707/95 (1307.Z.14/1 September 1890), BOA Ayniyat1024/181 (1286/1869–70), and BOA NGG 772/18 (1285. Ca.18/6 September 1868) for Medina; BOA İ.DH 601/41904 (1286.Ş.2/7 November 1869), BOA Ayniyat1028/209 (1286/1869–70), and BOA Ayniyat1024/202 (1286/1869–70) for Mecca; BOA İ.ŞD 26/1216 (1290.M.11/11 March 1873), BOA DH.MKT 1619/28 (1306.Ş.23/24 April 1889), BOA Ayniyat 1044/159 (1289/1872–3) for Erzurum; DH.MKT 1476/627 (1305.R.27/12 January 1888) for Kütahya and Eskişehir; BOA DH.MKT 1738/67 (1307.Za.14/2 July 1890) for Erzincan; BOA DH.MKT 1486/29 (1305.C.3/16 February 1888), BOA DH.MKT 1489/29 (1305.C.3/16 Febuary 1888), BOA DH.MKT 1490/9 (1305.C.15/28 February 1888) for Abha; BOA DH.MKT 1589/55 (1306.Ca.28/30 January 1889) for Basra, and BOA Ayniyat 1028/209 (1286/1869–70) are just a few such examples.
4. BOA A.MKT.UM 396/66 (1276.B.23/16 February 1860).
5. BOA A.MKT.DV 198/93 (1278.S.7/14 August 1861).

6. Although I checked the court registers of Kemer-i Edremit, I was not able to come up with this case, which led me to conclude that this case might have never been tried. Registers numbers are Burhaniye: 1101, 1103, Edremit: 1259, 1260, 1261.
7. BOA NGG 772/57 (1283.L.18/23 February 1867).
8. BOA DH.MKT 1924/67 1309 (1309.B.21/20 February 1892).
9. BOA DH.MKT 1802/28 (1308.C.13/24 January 1891) and BOA DH.MKT 1819/28 (1308.Ş.6/17 March 1891).
10. BOA Y.PRK.AZN 3/46 (1306.Ca.23/25 January 1889).
11. BOA DH.MKT 453/19 (1319.Z.7/17 March 1902).
12. Although, due to my emphasis on midwifery, I limited my attention to the reports of malpractice in this field, it is possible to find petitions in almost every field of medicine.
13. Ş. Kurnaz, *Cumhuriyet Öncesinde Türk Kadını: 1839–1923* (Ankara: Başbakanlık Aile Araştırma Kurumu, 1991); T. Oktar, *Osmanlı Toplumunda Kadının Çalışma Yaşamı: Osmanlı Kadınları Çalıştırma Cemiyet-i İslamiyesi* (Istanbul: Bilim Teknik Yayınevi, 1998).
14. Y. I. Ülman, 'Journal de Constantinople'a göre Mekteb-i Tıbbiye-i Adliye-i Şahane'nin Galatasaray Dönemi' (MA Thesis, Istanbul University, 1994); N. Sarı, 'Osmanlı Sağlık Hayatında Kadının Yeri', *New History of Medicine Studies*, 2–3 (1996–7), pp. 11–64; S. Bozkurt, 'Başlangıcından Günümüze İstanbul Tıp Fakültesinin Kadın Öğretim Üyeleri', in Yıldırım (ed.), *Sağlık Alanında Türk Kadını*, pp. 166–86; N. Sarı, 'Osmanlı Sağlık Hayatında Kadının Yerine Kısa bir Bakış', in *Sağlık Alanında Türk Kadını*; F. Saygılıgil, 'Osmanlı'da Sağlık Alanında Tedavi Gören ve Tedavi Eden Olarak Kadınlar', in A. İlyasoğlu and N. Akgökçe (eds), *Yerli Bir Feminizme Doğru* (Istanbul: Sel, 2001), pp. 127–54 in *Yerli Bir Feminizme Doğru* (Sel Yayıncılık, 2001); N. Yıldırım, 'Kadınların Hekim Olma Mücadelesi', *Toplumsal Tarih*, 147 (2006), pp. 50–7.
15. For critical evaluation of the dominance of this approach, see D. Harley, 'Historians as Demonologists: The Myth of the Midwife-Witch', *Social History of Medicine*, 3 (1990), pp. 1–26.
16. B. Ehrenreich and D. English, *Witches, Midwives and Nurses: A History of Women Healers* (New York, 1973); for a much more recent example of the same approach, see T. McIntosh, 'Profession, Skill, or Domestic Duty? Midwifery in Sheffield, 1881–1936', *Social History of Medicine*, 11:3 (1998), pp. 403–20. L. T. Ulrich, *A Midwife's Tale: The Life of Martha Ballard, Based on her Diary, 1785–1812* (New York: Knopf, 1990). For a challenging account, see M. H. Green, 'Gendering the History of Women's Healthcare', *Gender & History*, 20:3 (2008), pp. 487–518.
17. The articles in the volume edited by Hilary Marland are very good examples challenging the Anglo-Saxon model and searching for more complex dynamics in the changes in midwifery practices in Early Modern Europe. See H. Marland (ed.), *The Art of Midwifery: Early Modern Midwives in Europe* (London: Routledge, 1994). For another work that both criticizes this approach and offers an alternative, see A. M. Tuchman, '"The True Assistant to the Obstetrician": State Regulation and the Legal Protection of Midwives in Nineteenth Century Prussia', *Social History of Medicine*, 18:1 (2005), pp. 23–38. For non-Western critique of the same approach, see A. Homei, 'Sanba and their Clients: Midwives and the Medicalization of Childbirth in Japan', in B. Mortimer and S. McGann (eds), *New Directions in the History of Nursing* (London: Routledge, 2005), pp. 68–85; A. Homei, 'Birth Attendants in Meiji Japan: The Rise of a Medical Birth Model and the New Division of Labour', *Social History of Medicine*, 19:3 (2006), pp. 407–24.

18. For example, Wiesner shows that in Germany, although midwives could not be excluded from practice, they were placed under the control of male authorities, so as to show that they were not practising independently. In order to do that, the authorities kept midwives' public salaries low, placed them first under the control and scrutiny of 'honourable women' who did not have any medical expertise but the social and economic status to judge the functions of the midwives, and then gave the university trained physicians the right to approve midwives' licenses. M. Wiesner, 'The Midwives of South Germany and the Public/Private Dichotomy', in Marland, *The Art of Midwifery*, pp. 77–94. Lindemann's research also shows that the male practitioners/midwives in early modern Germany did not try to push the midwives away from but rather tried to intrude into and control their practices and redefine their tasks. Lindemann, 'Professionals? Sisters? Rivals?'
19. Tuchman; in the Middle Eastern context, Fahmy's work also confirms this approach. K. Fahmy, 'Women, Medicine and Power in Nineteenth-Century Egypt', in L. Abou-Lughod (ed.), *Remaking Women: Feminism and Mdoernity in the Middle East* (Princeton, NJ: Princton University Press, 1988), pp. 35–72.
20. D. Evenden, 'Mothers and their Midwives in the Seventeenth Century London', in Marland, *The Art of Midwifery*; D. Evenden, *The Midwives of Seventeenth Century London* (Cambridge University Press, 2000).
21. Harley, 'Provincial Midwives in England: 1660-1760', in Marland, *The Art of Midwifery*.
22. Lindemann, 'Professionals? Sisters? Rivals?'
23. I will concentrate on this issue more elaborately in Chapter 4.
24. S. Broomhall, '"Women's Little Secrets": Defining the Boundaries of Reproductive Knowledge in Sixteenth Century', *Social History of Medicine*, 15:1 (2002), pp. 1–15.
25. J. Bogdan, 'Care or Cure? Childbirth Practices in Nineteenth Century America', *Feminist Studies*, 4:2 (1978), pp. 92–9. N. S. Dye, 'History of Childbirth in America', *Signs*, 6:1, Women: Sex and Sexuality, Part 2 (1980), pp. 97–108. As Leavitt underlines, much of the experience of childbirth was controlled by pregnant and parturient women. Mostly they determined the setting of their births, the people who would attend them during labour and delivery, as well as the aids and comforts employed. In this scheme, the midwife was not interventionist but rather supportive of the parturient woman. J. W. Leavitt, '"Science" Enters the Birthing Room: Obstetrics in America since the Eighteenth Century', *Journal of American History*, 70:2 (1983), pp. 281–304; J. W. Leavitt, *Brought to Bed: Child Bearing in America, 1750–1950* (Oxford University Press, 1986).
26. A. C. Banks, *Birth Chairs, Midwives and Medicine* (Jackson, MS: University Press of Mississippi, 1999).
27. Schlumbohm, 'The Pregnant Women are Here for the Sake of the Teaching Institution', pp. 59–78.
28. Leavitt, '"Science" Enters the Birthing Room'; Dye, 'History of Childbirth in America'; M. Poovey, 'Scenes of an Indelicate Character: The Medical "Treatment" of Victorian Women', *Representations*, 14, *The Making of the Modern Body: Sexuality and Society in the Nineteenth Century* (1986), pp. 137–68.
29. L. T. Ulrich, '"The Living Mother of a Living Child": Midwifery and Mortality in Post-Revolutionary New England', *William and Mary Quarterly*, 46:1 (1989), pp. 27–48. I. Loudin, *Death in Childbirth: An International Study of Maternal Care and Maternal Mortality, 1800–1950* (Oxford, 1992); I. Loudin, 'Deaths in Childbed from the Eighteenth Century to 1935', *Medical History*, 30 (1986), pp. 1–41.
30. O. Moscucci, *The Science of Woman: Gynaecology and Gender in England, 1800–1929* (Cambridge University Press, 1990).

31. M. F. Hatem, 'The Professionalization of Health and the Control of Women's Bodies as Modern Governmentalities in Nineteenth-Century Egypt', in M. Zilfi *Women in the Ottoman Empire*.
32. Fahmy, 'Women, Medicine and Power'.
33. H. Abugideiri, 'The Scientisation of Culture: Colonial Medicine's Construction of Egyptian Womanhood, 1893–1929', *Gender and History*, 16:1 (2004), pp. 83–98; H. Abugideiri, 'Egyptian Women and the Science Question: Gender in the Making of Colonized Medicine, 1893–1929' (PhD dissertation, Georgetown University, 2001).
34. L. Kozma, *Policing Egyptian Women: Sex, Law, and Medicine in Khedival Egypt* (Syracuse, NY: Syracuse University Press, 2011).
35. Abdülaziz Bey (1850–1918) had written his renowned book, *Ottoman Customs, Ceremonies and Idioms*, around 1910s. Since Abdülaziz belonged to an elite family and built his career in some of the highest state offices, his account is limited to the customs and ceremonies that were practised among Muslim elites in the capital despite his claims of universality, which is also a common aspect of the genre. In addition to the opening chapter, Abdülaziz handled midwifery again in the section about health and medicine and gave the names of some of the most renowned and respectable midwives in contemporary Istanbul. Abdülaziz said that the midwives in the Ottoman society comprised three groups: *Saray-ı hümayun ebesi*, the midwife of the imperial harem; *kibar ebesi*, the midwife of the wealthy; and *ahad-ı nas ebesi*, the midwife of the common people. He described the first two groups in length, underlining that the first group was the most respectable of all and the second was also quite well off and respectable. It is not surprising that he said nothing about the third group at all. As such, his account also brings forward the social hierarchies in Ottoman society. See Abdülaziz, *Osmanlı Adet, Merasim ve Tabirleri/Adat ve Merasim-i Kadime, Tabirat ve Muamelat-i Kavmiye-i Osmaniye*, ed. K. Arısan and D. A. Günay (Istanbul: Tarih Vakfı Yurt Yayınları, 1995). For information on Abdülaziz, see M. Süreyya, *Sicill-i Osmani*, 6 vols (Istanbul: Tarih Vakfı Yurt Yayınları, 1996), and İbnü'l Emin Mahmut Kemal İnal, *Son Asır Türk Şairleri* (Istanbul: Türk Tarih Encümeni Külliyatı, 1930), pp. 44–7.
36. See, for example, BOA DH.MKT 1738/67 (1307.Za.14/2 July 1890), BOA DH.MKT 1444/73 (1304.Z.17/6 September 1887), BOA İ.DH 1057/82996 (1305.Ra.14/30 November 1887), BOA DH.MKT 1606/4 (1306.B.15/17 March 1889) for cases related to the midwives at Üsküdar police station.
37. Ülman, *Journal de Constantinople'a Göre*.
38. BOA HAT 827/37465 (3.Z.1253/28 February 1838), BOA HAT 1172/46356 (29.Z.1253/26 March 1838), BOA HAT 746/35262 (29.Z.1253/26 March 1838).
39. *Ceride-i Havadis*, Safer.18.1257/11 April 1841, no: 29.
40. Ibid.
41. BOA İ.MVL 44/830 (1258.N.11/17 September 1842).
42. Ibid.
43. The official documents persistently used the term 'science' rather than 'occupation' or 'field of expertise' in the place of midwifery, presumably to distinguish the knowledge provided in the school from the locally produced one.
44. One of the major contemporary journals, *Ceride-i Havadis*, also announced that a midwife from France, Madame Ventura, would be appointed at the School of Medicine in its building at Galatasaray in Beyoğlu district of the capital and assist difficult births without discriminating women along race or ethnicity. See *Ceride-i Havadis*, Safer.18.1257/11 April 184,1 no. 29.

45. BOA İ.MVL 44/830 (1258.N.11/17 September 1842).
46. The secondary data tells us that thirty-six women graduated from the courses, sixteen of whom were Christian. The sources indicate that Jewish midwives did not attend the courses. The literature assumes that Jewish midwives professionalized in abortion and take their absence from the midwifery courses as an evidence of this assumption arguing that they tried to hide themselves from government control. On these two issues see Kurnaz, *Cumhuriyet Öncesinde*; Oktar, *Osmanlı Toplumunda Kadının*; Ülman, *Journal de Constantinople*; and Taşkıran 'Türkiye'de Ebelik'.
47. BOA A.MKT.NZD 26/48 (1267.R.1/3 February 1851).
48. For some examples, see BOA A.MKT.MHM 222/10 (1277.Z.29/8 July 1861) and BOA A.MKT.MHM 366/35 (1278.Ra.4/9 September 1861) for Lesbos; BOA DH.MKT 1342/92 (1301.S.24/25 December 1883), BOA DH.MKT 1517/98 (1305.L.20/30 June 1888), and BOA DH.MKT 1538/25 (1305.Z.22/ 30 August 1888) for Erzurum; BOA DH.MKT 1622/47 (1306.N.9/9 May1889) for Beirut; BOA DH.MKT 1628/59 (1306.L.14/13 June 1889) for Çatalca; BOA DH.MKT 1435/86 (1304. Za.11/1 August 1887) for Bagdad; BOA DH.MKT 624/43 (1320.Ş.29/1 December 1902); and BOA DH.MKT 711/66 (1321.S.22/ 20 May 1903) for Damascus.
49. For some examples, see BOA MV 30/3 (1305.B.2/15 March 1888); BOA A.MKT. NZD 315/39 (1276.Za.29/18 June 1860); BOA DH.MKT 1516/59 (1305.L.16/26 June 1888); BOA DH.MKT 1573/33 (1306.R.6/10 December 1888); BOA DH.MKT 1616/100 (1306.Ş.15/16 April 1889); BOA DH.MKT 1412/13 (1304.B.29/23 April 1887); BOA DH.MKT 1435/86 (1304.Za.11/1 August 1887); BOA DH.MKT 1408/29 (1304.B.5/30 March 1887); BOA DH.MKT 1538/25 (1305.Z.22/30 August 1888); BOA DH.MKT 1363/108 (1303.Z.7/6 September 1886); BOA DH.MKT 1353/84 (1303.L.5/7 July 1886).
50. For one such example, see BOA DH.MKT 510/57(1320.S.15/ 24 May 1902). Here it is ordered that the unlicensed surgeons, dentists, pharmacists and the midwives in Monastir should be punished by fines, sent to the School of Medicine to take licenses and finally their names should be denounced in local newspapers. This document is interesting in terms of demonstrating the change of the means to impose the government will and it also confirms that the government's real concern was not about the skill or capability of the midwives or other medical professionals, but about licensing and regulating them. This example also demonstrates that the development of the published media did also mean the introduction of novel and efficient methods of control.
51. Check for 'Memalik-i Mahruse-i Şahanede Tababet-i Belediyye İcrasına Dair Nizamname', in Osman Nuri Ergin, *Mecelle-i Umur-u Belediyye*, 6 vols (Istanbul: İstanbul Büyükşehir Belediyesi Kültür İşleri Daire Başkanlığı, 1995), vol. 6, p. 3053.
52. The major focus related to midwifery was about foreign midwives and the procedure to be followed in order to receive proper licenses. In order to do that, they needed first to have their passports approved and signed by the embassies of their home countries. After that, they would take an exam at the School of Medicine, and those who passed the exam would pay one hundred *guruş* to receive their licenses. Those who worked in the provinces should have a copy of their licenses approved by the consulates of their countries and send this copy to the Directorate of the School of Medicine through the provincial governor. I also want to note that according to this regulation, doctors or surgeons paid five hundred *guruş*, five times more than the midwives. This is in conformity with similar documents, which mention the mediocre financial means of the midwives compared to doctors and pharmacists, and that they should be supported by the state.

This policy was also a strategy to encourage a higher number of midwives to be registered and licensed. For information about foreign midwives opening private offices in Ottoman lands, which was a rather common phenomena, see also Yıldırım, 'Kadınların Hekim Olma Mücadelesi', pp. 50–7.

53. BOA DH.MKT 1343/10 (1301.S.26/27 December 1883). Unfortunately I was unable to cross-check this document from the Council of State classifications, since the Prime Ministry Archive does not hold the complete collection. The document I used was a copy reproduced by the Ministry of the Interior upon the communication of the Council of State.
54. See Chapter 3 for a detailed discussion of this issue.
55. BOA Cevdet Sıhhiye, 13/650 (1264.M.20/28 December 1847).
56. In such documents, the term obstetrician is almost never used and rather the term 'doctor skilled in obstetrics' (*Fenn-i kıbalede mahirettıba*) is preferred presumably due to the low number of obstetricians of that period.
57. BOA DH.MKT 1343/10 (1301.S.26/27 December 1883).
58. BOA DH.MKT 1343/10 (1301.S.26/27 December 1883).
59. This document was sent to almost all provincial centers such as Edirne, Aydın, Hicaz, Bagdad, Salonika, Diyarbakır, Aleppo, Tripoli, Sivas, Monastir, İşkodra, Mamuratülaziz, Van, Yanya and Mosul.
60. BOA DH.MKT 1573/33 (1306.R.6/10 December 1888).
61. For some quick replies see BOA DH.MKT 1619/126 (1306.Ş.26/27 April 1889) from Çatalca, Silivri, Terkos; BOA DH.MKT 1620/89 (1306.Ş.29/30 April 1889) from Biga; BOA DH.MKT 1630/110 (1306.L.24/23 June 1889) from Kos, and BOA DH.MKT 1396/18 (1304.Ca.5/30 January 1887) from Aleppo. These places sent lists containing the names, ages and the types of the licenses of the medical workers in the town.
62. BOA DH.MKT 1441/41 (1304.Z.1/21 August 1887) and BOA DH.MKT 1400/1(1304.Ca.22/16 February 1887).
63. BOA DH.MKT 1408/29 (1304.B.05/30 March 1887).
64. BOA DH.MKT 1463/15 (1305.S.27/14 November 1887).
65. BOA DH.MKT 1475/50 (1305.R.21/6 January 1888).
66. BOA HR.TO 263/88 (1888.8.11).
67. BOA HR.TO 143/87 (1887.11.22).
68. BOA HR.TO 167/127 (1889.3.8).
69. BOA DH.MKT 1472/49 (1305.R.12/28 December 1887).
70. BOA DH.MKT 1532/96 (1305.Z.6/14 August 1888).
71. BOA DH.MKT 1465/3 (1305.Ra.5/21 November 1887).
72. BOA DH.MKT 1520/35(1305.L.28/8 July 1888).
73. For a set of documents that demonstrate this internal negotiation and cooperation, see BOA DH.MKT 1531/101 (1305.Z.4/12 August 1888); BOA DH.MKT 1561/6 (1306.Ra.1/5 November 1888); BOA DH.MKT 1564/56 (1306.Ra.17/21 November 1888); BOA DH.MKT 1568/80 (1306.Ra.22/26 November 1888); BOA DH.MKT 1579/97 (1306.R.25/29 December 1888); and BOA DH.MKT 1585/18 (1306.Ca.15/17 January 1889).
74. BOA DH.MKT 1506/7 (1305.Ş.21/3 May 1888) and BOA DH.MKT 1506/49 (1305.Ş.22/4 May 1888).
75. BOA DH.MKT 1536/113 (1305.Z.20/28 August 1888).
76. BOA DH.MKT 1559/54 (1306.S.24/30 October 1888) and BOA DH.MKT 2087/50 (1315.B.23/18 December 1897).

77. BOA DH.MKT 2089/57 (1316.M.2/23 May 1898) and BOA DH.MKT 2173/30 (1316.L.19/2 March 1899).
78. BOA DH.MKT 1549/71 (1306.M.25/1 October 1888).
79. BOA DH.MKT 1976/38 (1309.Z.27/23 July 1892).
80. BOA DH.MKT 1989/89 (1310.M.25/19 August 1892), DH.MKT 2004/99 1310.S.29/22 September 1892).
81. BOA DH.MKT 59/30 (1311.B.27/3 February 1894), Annex 1.
82. BOA DH.MKT 59/30 (1311.B.27/3 February 1894), Annex 2.
83. BOA DH.MKT 59/30 (1311.B.27/3 February 1894), Annex 3.
84. BOA DH.MKT 59/30 (1311.B.27/3 February 1894), Annex 4.
85. BOA DH.MKT 59/30 (1311.B.27/3 February 1894), Annex 6.
86. BOA DH.MKT 59/30 (1311.B.27/3 February 1894), Annex 5.
87. BOA DH.MKT 59/30 (1311.B.27/3 February 1894), Annex 7.
88. BOA DH.MKT 59/30 (1311.B.27/3 February 1894), Annex 8.
89. BOA DH.MKT 236/34 (1311.Za.10/15 May 1894).
90. BOA DH.MKT 339/27 (1312.Ş.5/1 February 1895).
91. BOA DH.MKT 295/77 (1312.R.15/16 October 1895).
92. BOA A.MKT.NZD 315/39 (1276.Za.29/18 June 1860); The licensed midwife Neblevi was appointed to Haseki Women's hospital BOA DH.MKT 76/47 (1310.Z.18/3 July 1893); Refika hanım who was a graduate of the Midwifery School was appointed to the *Bimarhane* BOA DH.MKT 1997/16 (1310.S.13/6 September 1892); Vangelice was appointed to Üsküp BOA DH.MKT 23/50 (1311.S.2/15 August 1993), however, for some reason only two years later she asked her appointment to Adana from Üsküp BOA DH.MKT 331/16 (1312.B.13/10 January 1895); the midwife Oniko was appointed to Haseki Women's Hospital BOA DH.MKT 319/30 and BOA DH.MKT 341/2 (1312.Ş.9/5 February 1895); the licensed midwife Maryam Magagyan asked for an appointment BOA DH.MKT 372/10 (1312.Za.12/7 May 1895); midwife Emetullah was appointed to Jerusalem BOA DH.MKT 2099/120 (1316.R.14/1 September 1898); the appointment of midwife Pinopi Dimitriyo either in Haseki Women's Hospital or some other location BOA DH.MKT 103/4 (1311.M.22/ 5 August 1893); the licensed midwife Yani who was living in Balat asked her appointment BOA DH.MKT 379/21 (1312.Z.2/27 May 1895); Madame Apyar told that she was willing to assist the births at the Darülaceze if her travel expenses were covered BOA DH.MKT 583/48 (1320.C.22/26 September 1902); for the appointment of Emine hanım BOA NGG 772/34 (1283.C.24/3 November 1866); midwife Hatice hanım was appointed to Mecca BOA NGG 772/17 (1286.C.21/28 September 1869).
93. Midwife Madame Liza requested appointment to the position at the Police Department, but unfortunately replied negatively since there was no such opening BOA DH.MKT 1566/79 (1306.Ra.17/ 21 November 1888) and BOA DH.MKT 1593/26 (1306.C.10/11 February 1889); Eliza was rejected BOA DH.MKT 2091/17 (1316. Ra.26/13 September 1898); midwife Sarine's request for appointment to Salonika was rejected since she failed the exam BOA DH.MKT 441/47 (1319.Z.5/15 March 1902).
94. The Erzincan midwife Zinte Hanım was granted a salary BOA DH.MKT 197/3 (1311.B.10/17 January 1894); midwife Eliza who was voluntarily assisting birth in Kuzguncuk, Istanbul asked the Ministry of Interior for a wage, and her proposal was approved BOA DH.MKT 2054/14 (1310.Ş.3/20 February 1893); the midwife of Hama and Humus, Huriye Şerife Hanım sent a petition to the Ministry of the Interior asking for her unpaid salaries and they responded positively BOA DH.MKT 2098/46

(1316.R.12/30 August 1898); the midwives Fatma Hanım and Nefise Hanım asked to receive monetary payment rather than food allowance, and their pledge was accepted İ.DH 496/33692 (1279.Ra.13/8 September 1862); BOA DH.MKT 746/87 (1321. Ca.9/3 August 1903) ordered the regular payment of the salaries of several midwives at different locations. Ayşe Hanım who was voluntarily assisting childbirths in Üsküdar, Istanbul was granted a salary BOA ZB 77/7 (1302.N.24/7 July 1885); Naile Hanım was granted a salary BOA NGG 772 (1289.Ş.21/24 October 1872); midwife Kamer Hanım was granted a wage of 1000 *guruş* BOA NGG 772/3 (1290.M.17/17 February 1873).

95. BOA DH.MKT 1582/100 (1306.Ca.7/9 January 1889).
96. BOA DH.MKT 506/19 (1320.S.9/18 May 1902).
97. The Ministry of Interior ordered the regular payment of the salaries of the midwives BOA DH.MKT 2089/57 (1316.M.2/23 May 1898); Hafiza Hanım, the midwife of Medina asked her due payments BOA DH.MKT 1621/124 (1306.N.7/7 May 1889) and BOA DH.MKT 2189/17 (1316.Z.1/12 April 1899); midwife Naile of the School of Medicine asked for an increase in her salary BOA Ayniyat 1034/136 (1296/1878–9); midwife Naile Hanım asked for an increase BOA NGG 772/30 (1292.L.21/20 November 1875) and BOA NGG 771/27 (1289.Ş.27/30 October 1872).
98. BOA HR.MKT 71/40 (1263.S.16/3.2.1847).
99. For some such cases, see BOA NGG 772/24 (1278.Ca.13/16 November 1861), BOA NGG 772/58 (1278.R.25/30 October 1861), and BOA A.MKT.NZD 417/94 (1278. Za.13/12 May 1862) and for Inrit Roberts; BOA HR.MKT 17/40 (1263.S.16/3 February 1847) for Marya; and BOA DH.MKT 669/36 (1320.Z.20/20 March 1903) for Anastasya Kaloyanini.
100. BOA DH.MKT 295/77 (1312.R.15/12 January 1895); BOA DH.MKT 154/18 (1311.R.9/20 September 1893).
101. BOA DH.MKT 2173/30 (1316.L.19/2 March 1899).
102. For example, Madame Mesati received retirement pension after she quit practising midwifery due to her old age; after her death, her two daughters applied to continue receiving her pension and their application was successful and received quite positively. See BOA İ.DH 145/7498 (1263.Ca.10/26 April 1847), BOA HR.MKT 40/80 (1268.S.22/17 December 1851), and BOA HR.MKT 42/89 (1268.R.16/8 January 1852).
103. BOA İ.DH 1057/82996 (1305.Ra.14/30 November 1887) The midwife of Üsküdar, Ayşe; BOA İ.DH 927/73500 (1301.Za.16/7 October 1884) midwife Madame Liza again of Üsküdar; BOA İ.DH 1274/100155 (1309.L.6/44 May 1892) midwife Revirsemi of the School of Medicine; BOA İ.HR 193/5889 (1267.S.10/15 Demember 1850) midwife Anata of the School of Medicine; BOA İ.TAL 26 /1311.M.71 (1311.M.18/1 August 1893) Emine Hanım known as the Civan ebe; BOA İ.TAL 107/1314.B.2 (1314.B.1/6 December 1896) Şakire Hanım who was the midwife of Medine; BOA İ.TAL 129/1315.N.97 (1315.N.26/1 February 1898) midwife Emine Tevhide Hanım; BOA Y.A.RES 103/26 (1317.Ca.14/20 September 1899) Marice are some of the examples.
104. For example, BOA DH.MKT 1427/99 (1304.L.7/29 June 1887) is about the appointment of a certain midwife Muhsine Hanım; BOA DH.MKT 59/30 (1311.B.27/3 February 1894) is about midwife Nefise.
105. BOA DH.MKT 1503.67 (1305.Ş.12/24 April 1888).
106. BOA DH.MKT 372/10 (1312.Za.12/7 May 1895); another example of a repair request BOA A.MKT.NZD 35/98 (1267.Ş.4/4 June 1851).

107. BOA DH.MKT 1996/40 (1309.S.11/16 September 1891), BOA Y.PRK.ASK 176/45 (1319.B.10/23 Otocber 1901).
108. BOA DH.MKT 401/61 (1313.S.2/24 July 1895).
109. Here the Ladino term 'komadre' was used.
110. *El Messeret*, 25 June 1897, p. 173. A systematic research through the contemporary newspapers would uncover many similar announcements. I am grateful to Nazan Maksudyan for bringing this document to my attention.
111. *Hanımlara Mahsus Gazete*, 10.L.1315/4 March 1898, no. 151. For another example see, A. Basiretçi, 'Şehir Mektubu, no. 157', *Basiret*, 2318 (13.Ra.1295/17 January 1878), pp. 2–3. For the reprint, see A. E. Basiretçi, 'Kadın Ebeler (Kabileler)', in N. Sağlam, *İstanbul Mektupları* (Istanbul: Kitabevi, 2001), pp. 679–80.
112. 'İki Ebe Bir Gebe', *Hayâl-i Cedîd*, 55–60 (28 October 1910–18 November 1910). I am deeply grateful to Seval Şahin for bringing this vaudeville to my attention.
113. E. H. Fazıl, *Zenanname* (Istanbul Üniversitesi Library, 5502, 1206 (1791–2)), p. 142a.
114. BOA Cevdet Sıhhiye 13/650 (1264.M.20/29 December 1847). The most comprehensible account on this hospital is N. Taşkıran, *Haseki'nin Kitabı: İstanbul Haseki Külliyesi* (İstanbul: Haseki Hastanesini Kalkındırma Derneği, 1972).
115. For example, Schlumbohm, 'The Pregnant Women are Here for the Sake of the Teaching Institution', pp. 59–78.
116. BOA İ.ŞD 16/690 (1286.Ca.1/9 August 1869), BOA Ayniyat 1025/50 (1286.Ca.14/22 August 1869), and BOA NGG 772/13 (1286.Ca.15/23 August 1869).
117. The Istanbul municipality (*Şehremaneti*) inspected the construction site in 1870 and reported that an amount of 36.819 *guruş* was spent until then. BOA Ayniyat 1044/3 (1287.B/October 1870).
118. BOA İ.DH 652/45367 (1289.R.21/28 June 1872).
119. BOA NGG 771/17 (1289.C.8/13 August 1872), BOA Ayniyat 1033/197 (1297.S/January 1880), and BOA NGG 771/42 (1289.Ca.24/30 July 1872).
120. BOA NGG 771/23 (1289.B.19/22 September 1872).
121. BOA A.MKT.MHM 445/65 (1289.Za.16/15 January 1873).
122. BOA A.MKT.MHM 452/14 (1290.S.14/13 April 1873).
123. BOA NGG 771/36 (1292.M.3/9 February 1875).
124. BOA Ayniyat 1033/197/ (1297.S/January 1880).
125. BOA DH.MKT 1396/122 (1304.Ca.7/1 February 1887) and BOA DH.MKT 1466/13/ (1305.Ra.11/27 November 1887). A non-Muslim Ottoman woman called Elena wanted to donate her land in Beyoğlu district to the Ottoman government on the condition of the construction of a maternity clinic/midwifery school on it.
126. BOA İ.ŞD 77/4555/ (1303/1885–6).
127. BOA DH.MKT 2006/97 (1310.Ra.10/2 September 1892), BOA DH.MKT 2039/15 (1310.C.15/4 January 1893).
128. Besim Ömer, *Doğum Tarihi* (Istanbul: Ahmet İhsan Matbaası, 1932), p. 50.
129. Ibid, p. 51.
130. Ibid.
131. BOA DH.MKT 2039/15 (1310.C.15/4 January 1893).
132. BOA İ.HUS 21/1311.Ş.118 (1311.Ş.16 /21 February 1894).
133. BOA İ.DH 1338/1314.Ra.44 (1314.Ra.28/6 September 1896), BOA DH.MKT 558/25 (1320.Ca.7/12 September 1902).
134. BOA İ.ŞE 6/6 (1321.Ra.15/11 January 1903).
135. BOA ZB 322/8 (1323.Kanunsani.27/9 February 1908).

136. See N. Maksudyan, '"This Time Women as Well Got Involved in Politics!": Nineteenth Century Ottoman Women's Organizations and Political Agency', in S. Aprahamian and V. Rowe (eds),*Ottoman Women's Movements and Print Cultures* (Austin, TX: University of Texas Press, forthcoming).
137. BOA ZB 325/28 (1324.Kanunevvel.15/28 December 1908).
138. Ibid.
139. For some examples, see BOA DH.MKT 1444/73 (1304.Z.17/6 September 1887), BOA Y.PRK.AZJ 42/85 (1319.Ca.14/29 August 1901), and BOA Y.PRK.ASK 176/45 (1319.B.10/23 October 1901).
140. BOA DH.MKT 242/70 (1311.Za.24/29 May 1894).

3 Abortion, Power and Agency

1. BOA A.MKT.MHM 300/48 (1280.Z.8/15 May 1864).
2. BOA A.MKT.MHM 300/48 (1280.Z.8/15 May 1864).
3. The document used the term the 'kazahat', which means 'misdemeanor'.
4. BOA A.MKT.MHM 300/48 (1280.Z.8/15 May 1864).
5. BOA A.MKT.MHM 300/48 (1280.Z.8/15 May 1864).
6. C. Usborne, 'Abortion for Sale! The Competition between Quacks and Doctors in Weimar Germany', in M. Gijswit-Hofstra, H. Marland and Hans de Vaard (eds), *Illness and Healing Alternatives in Western Europe* (London: Routledge, 1997), pp. 183–204.
7. Kozma, *Policing Egyptian Women*; Green, 'Gendering the History of Women's Healthcare', pp. 487–518; J. E. Pedersen, 'Regulating Abortion and Birth Control: Gender, Medicine, and Republican Politics in France, 1870–1920', *French Historical Studies*, 19:3 (1996), pp. 673–98.
8. A. Grossman, *Reforming Sex: The German Movement For Birth Control and Abortion Reform 1920–1950* (New York: Oxford University Press, 1995); U. Rublack, 'The Public Body: Policing Abortion in Early Modern Germany', in L. Abrams and E. Harvey (eds), *Gender Relations in German History: Power, Agency, and Experience from the Sixteenth to the Twentieth Century* (Durham, NC: Duke University Press, 1997), pp. 57–80. C. Usborne, 'Wise Women, Wise Men and Abortion in the Weimar Republic: Gender, Class and Medicine', in Abrams and Harvey (eds), *Gender Relations in German History*, pp. 143–76. See also the parts on abortion in L. Engelstein, *The Keys to Happiness: Sex and the Search for Modernity in Fin-de-siècle Russia* (Ithaca, NY: Cornell University Press, 1992).
9. A. McLaren, 'Abortion in France: Women and the Regulation of Family Size, 1800–1914', *French Historical Studies*, 10:3 (Spring 1978), pp. 461–85; A. McLaren, 'Abortion in England, 1890-1914', *Victorian Studies* 20/4 (1977), pp. 379–401; A. McLaren, *Reproductive Rituals: The Perception of Fertility in England from the Sixteenth to the Nineteenth Century* (London: Methuen, 1984) also addresses the problem.
10. For example, see M. Oztürk, 'Osmanlı Döneminde Iskat-ı Cenin Yeri ve Hükmü', *Fırat Üniversitesi Dergisi (Sosyal Bilimler)*, 1:1 (1987), pp. 199–208. K. Olgun, 'Osmanlı Devletinde Nüfusu Arttırma Politikası Çerçevesinde Iskat-ı Ceninin (Kürtaj) Yasaklanması', *Uluslararası Tıp Tarihi Kongresi*, 38 (2002: Ankara), ed. N. Sarı (Ankara: Türk Tarih Kurumu, 2005). Duben and Behar, *Istanbul Households*. For a recent work, see F. Simşek, H. Eroğlu and G. Dinç 'Osmanlı İmparatorluğunda Iskat-ı Cenin (Çocuk Düşürme)', in *Uluslararası Sosyal Araştırmalar Dergisi/ Journal of International Social Research*, 2:6 (Winter 2009), pp. 593–609.

11. One example to the works that have a long term approach is A. Gürsoy, 'Abortion in Turkey: A Matter of State, Family or Individual Decision', *Social Science and Medicine*, 42:4 (1996), pp. 531–42. Gürsoy first discusses briefly the 1858 criminal code and then extends her account from the early Republican periods to the present. Another example of this approach can be found in D. L. Bowen, 'Abortion, Islam, and the 1994 Cairo Population Conference', *International Journal of Middle East Studies*, 29:2 (1997), pp. 161–84.
12. S. A. Somel, 'Osmanlı Son Döneminde Iskat-ı Cenin Meselesi', *Kebikeç*, 13 (2002), pp. 65–88; S. A. Somel, 'The Issue of Abortion in 19th Century Ottoman Empire', in H. İnalcık and O. Özel (eds), *IXth International Congress of Economic and Social History of Turkey Dubrovnik-Croatia, 20–23 August, 2002* (Ankara: Atatürk Supreme Council for Culture, Language & History Publications of the Turkish Historical Society, 2005), pp. 339–46.
13. T. Demirci and S. A. Somel, 'Women's Bodies, Demography, and Public Health: Abortion Policy and Perspectives in the Ottoman Empire of the Nineteenth Century', *Journal of the History of Sexuality*, 17:3 (2008), pp. 377–420.
14. R. Miller, *The Limits of Bodily Integrity: Abortion, Adultery, and Rape Legislation in Comparative Perspective* (Aldershot: Ashgate, 2007); R. Miller, 'Politicizing Reproduction in Comparative Perspective: Ottoman, Turkish, and French Approaches to Abortion Law', *Hawwa*, 5:1 (2007), pp. 73–89; R. Miller, 'Rights, Reproduction, Sexuality, and Citizenship in the Ottoman Empire and Turkey', *Signs*, 32:2 (Winter 2007), pp. 347–75.
15. For example, Rublack draws her work on abortion on sixty two cases brought before south-west German courts. See Rublack, 'The Public Body'.
16. Usborne bases her research on cases including police interviews and pre-trial investigations as well as the interrogations during the main trial. Usborne, 'Wise Women, Wise Men'.
17. McLaren, 'Abortion in France'.
18. BOA A.M 18/80 (1275.M.07/17 July 1858).
19. The contemporary dictionaries also give both meanings of the term, for example, in Sir J. W. Redhouse's *Turkish and English Lexicon*, the term *ıskat-ı cenin* is translated as both abortion and miscarriage, whereas Şemseddin Sami's well-respected *Kamus-ı Türki* explains *ıskat-ı cenin* as purposefully dropping a baby from the uterus, or the crime of allowing an abortion (*rahimden kasden çocuk düşürmek veya düşürtmek cinayeti*). See Sir J. W. Redhouse, *Turkish and English Lexicon* (London: Oriental Literature Society, 1309 (1892)) and Şemseddin Sami, *Kamus-ı Türki, I* (Dersaadet: İkdam Matbaası, 1317 (1899)).
20. For example, Ahmet Akgündüz in his widely referred book which is an introduction to court records specifies *ıskat-ı cenin* (meaning miscarriage) as a subcategory of murder crimes and gives an example from the sixteenth century. A. Akgündüz, *Şer'iye Sicilleri: Mahiyeti, Toplu Kataloğu ve Seçme Hükümler* (Istanbul: Türk Dünyası Araştırmaları Vakfı, 1988). For the legal approaches to intentionally causing a miscarriage, see C. Imber, *Ebu's-Su'ud: The Islamic Legal Tradition* (Stanford, CA: Stanford University Press, 1997), p. 239.
21. Somel, 'Osmanlı Son Döneminde Iskat-ı Cenin'; Demirci and Somel, 'Women's Bodies'; Bowen, 'Abortion, Islam'. See also, J. E. Brockopp, *Islamic Ethics of Life: Abortion, War, and Euthanasia* (University of South Carolina Press, 2003). Specifically, see M. H. Katz, 'The Problem of Abortion in Classical Sunni Fikh', and Bowen in this volume.
22. The Supreme Council for Judicial Ordinances was an upper legislative council that discussed and prepared the necessary laws and regulations promised by the Tanzimat, and checked the implementation of these laws. For a more detailed discussion, see Akyıldız, *Tanzimat Dönemi Osmanlı Merkez*, pp. 189–217, and also Findley, *Bureaucratic Reform*, pp. 175–6.

23. The Council of the Sublime Porte was bureaucratically placed just below the Sublime Council for Judicial Ordinances and discussed and decided the legislation required prepared it and proposed it to the Sublime Council. See Akyıldız, *Tanzimat Dönemi Osmanlı Merkez*, pp. 218–21.
24. The Council of Public Works (Meclis-i Umur-u Nafia) was responsible for developing strategies regarding the economic and agricultural development as well as raising the welfare and prosperity of the country. See Akyıldız, *Tanzimat Dönemi Osmanlı Merkez*, pp. 258–64.
25. For the earlier attempts to ban abortion, see BOA Cevdet Sıhhiye 1026 (N.1204/April 1790), and BOA Cevdet Adliye 108 (1204.L.9/22 June 1790). See also BOA Cevdet Sıhhiye 9/437 (1242.Ş.12/11 March 1827). This document tells that a midwife, Polise, the daughter of Ahpa, was exiled to Salonika in 1827 for procuring abortifacients. The literature on abortion have frequently quoted this document as evidence that Jewish midwifes were known as 'bloodstained' midwives and were experts in abortion. The reproduction of this prejudiced stereotype also deserves a separate analysis.
26. 'Meclis-i Umur-u Nafianın Layihası', *Takvim-i Vekayi* (1254.Ş.28/16 November 1838). This document was also later been reprinted in the semi-official document collection. For this copy *Muharrerat-ı Nadire* (Istanbul, 1289 (1872)), pp. 750–2.
27. 'Meclis-i Umur-u Nafianın Layihası', *Takvim-i Vekayi* (1254.Ş.28/1 November 1838).
28. See, for example, BOA Cevdet Dahiliye 3225 (1254.N.13/30 November 1838); BOA Cevdet Dahiliye 51/2519 (1254.L.15/1 January 1839) for Üsküp; BOA Cevdet Sıhhiye 7/306 (1254.L.25/11 January 1839) for Rumeli; BOA BOA Cevdet Dahiliye 131/6543 (1254.Za.3/18 January 1839) for Niğde; Cevdet Dahiliye 36/1790 (1254.Za.5/20 January 1839) for Vize; BOA Cevdet Sıhhiye 12/566 (1254.Z.13/27 February 1839) for Babadağ; BOA Cevdet Dahiliye 136/6794 (1254.Z.19/5 March 1839) for İskenderiye.
29. 'Husus-u Mezbure Dair Dar-Şura-yı Bab-ı Aliden Yazılan Mazbata', *Takvim-i Vekayi*, 1254.Ş.28/16 November 1838. See also *Muharrerat-ı Nadire* (Istanbul: İzzet Efendi Matbaası, 1289/1872), pp. 753–4.
30. BOA A.DVN.NMH 2/15 (1254.Ş.25/13 November 1838).
31. BOA Cevdet Adliye 14/896 (1254.N.23/10 December 1838), BOA Cevdet Adliye 94/5849 (1254.L.27/13 January 1839). For a few examples, see see BOA Cevdet Dahiliye 3225 (1254.N.13/30 November 1838); BOA Cevdet Dahiliye 51/2519 (1254.L.15/1 January 1839) for Üsküp; BOA Cevdet Sıhhiye 7/306 (1254.L.25/11 January 1839) for Rumeli; BOA BOA Cevdet Dahiliye 131/6543 (1254.Za.3/18 January 1839) for Niğde; Cevdet Dahiliye 36/1790 (1254.Za.5/20 January 1839) for Vize; BOA Cevdet Sıhhiye 12/566 (1254.Z.13/27 February 1839) for Babadağ; BOA Cevdet Dahiliye 136/6794 (1254.Z.19/5 March 1839) for İskenderiye.
32. '*mügayir-i rıza-ı cenab-ı hallak-ı alem ve badi katl-i nesl-i benî Adem olan ıskat-ı cenin madde-i kerihesi*'.
33. 1.Rebiyülevvel.1256.
34. See the section about the Criminal code in A. Akgündüz, *Mukayeseli İslam ve Osmanlı Hukuku Külliyatı* (Diyarbakır: Dicle Üniversitesi Hukuk Fakültesi Yayınları, 1986), pp. 803–31. Demirci and Somel, 'Women's Bodies' also emphasize this point. See also Öztürk, 'Osmanlı Döneminde Iskat-ı Cenin', p. 201; T. Taner, 'Tanzimat Devrinde Ceza Hukuku', in *Tanzimat I* (Istanbul, 1940), pp. 226–30.
35. Demirci and Somel explain this hiatus with the return to Islamic values in this period. They argue that as a result of this return, abortion was not covered under modern laws. See Demirci and Somel, 'Women's Bodies'.
36. BOA İ.MVL 175/5190 (1266.Ş.22/3 July 1850).

37. It is important to remember that the Ottoman government required the shopkeepers to stand surety for another shopkeeper he knew as a measure for keeping the workforce under supervision. Here the guarantor refers to this kind of surety. For detailed information on this issue see C. Kırlı, 'A Profile of the Labor Force in Early Nineteenth-Century Istanbul', *International Labor and Working Class History*, 60 (2001), pp. 125–40.
38. '*Madde 192: Bir kimse darp yahut sair gune bir fil ile bir hamile hatunun ıskat-ı cenin eylemesine sebep olur ise, diyet-i şeriyesi istifa olunduktan sonra, eğer bu teaddisi an kasdin olmuş ise muvakkaten küreğe konulur.*
Madde 193: Bir hamile hatunun gerek rızası olsun ve gerek rızası olmasın iskat-ı cenin ettirmek için ilaç içirip yahut esbab ve vesailini tariff edip de eseriyle çocuğu düşürülür ise, buna sebep olan kimse altı aydan iki seneye kadar hapis olunur. Ve eğer buna sebep olan tabip ve cerrah ve eczacı ise muvakkaten küreğe konulur.' For a copy of the law in modern Turkish script see A. Akgündüz, Mukayeseli İslam ve Osmanlı Hukuku, p. 864.
The 1858 Criminal code was almost a mot-a-mot translation of the 1810 French Penal Code. See article 317: 'Quiconque, par aliments, breuvages, médicaments, violences, ou par tout autre moyen, aura procuré l'avortement d'une femme enceinte, soit qu'elle y ait consenti ou non, sera puni de la réclusion.
La même peine sera prononcée contre la femme qui se sera procuré l'avortement à elle-même, ou qui aura consenti à faire usage des moyens à elle indiqués ou administrés à cet effet, si l'avortement s'en est ensuivi.
Les médecins, chirurgiens et autres officiers de santé, ainsi que les pharmaciens qui auront indiqué ou administré ces moyens, seront condamnés à la peine des travaux forcés à temps, dans le cas où l'avortement aurait eu lieu.'
39. The Doctor's Association was founded in 1856. It was the first doctor's organization in the Ottoman Empire. It included both Muslim and non-Muslim Ottoman doctors, as well as some foreign ones. Besides playing a major role in the administration of medicine and public health, the Doctor's Association was the major advocate of licensing the doctors, pharmacists and the midwives. See also BOA İ.MVL 567/15500 (1283.L.25/2 March 1867).
40. BOA HR.TO 432/26 (1859.5.1).
41. BOA HR.TO 432/26 (1859.5.1).
42. For some of the examples of the stipends offered to those who took care of the foundlings, see BOA İ.MVL 141/3927 (1265.C.28/21 March 1849), BOA İ.MVL 228/7822 (1268.Ra.16/9 January 1852), BOA İ.MVL 290/11567 (1270.S.18/20 November 1853), BOA İ.MVL 304/12466 (1270.B.26/ 24 April 1854), BOA İ.MVL 313/13122 (1270.Z.3/27 August 1854), BOA İ.MVL 290/11567 (1270.S.28/30 November 1853), BOA İ.MVL 141/3927 (1265.C.28/ 21 Match 1849), BOA İ.MVL 228/7822 (1268. Ra.16/9 January 1852). See also N. Maksudyan, 'Hearing the Voiceless – Seeing the Invisible: Orphans and Destitute Children as Actors of Social, Economic, and Political History in the Late Ottoman Empire' (PhD Dissertation, Sabancı University, 2008).
43. BOA HR.TO 432/26 (1859 May).
44. It is possible to find a great number of such documents that document the requests and offer of financial aid for both Muslims and non-Muslims. For just a very few examples see BOA İ.MVL 310/12974 (1270.Za.1/26 July 1854), BOA İ.MVL 312/13056 (1270.Za.18/12 August 1854), BOA İ.MVL 313/13125 (1270.Z.3/27 August 1854), BOA İ.MVL 313/12127 (1270.Z.3/27 August 1854), BOA İ.MVL 320/13562 (1271. Ra.6/27 November 1854), BOA İ.MVL 337/14552 (1271.Za.28/12 August 1855), BOA A.MKT.NZD 143/100 (1271.B.24/12 April 1855), BOA A.MKT.NZD 159/56

(1271.Z.21/4 September 1855), BOA A.MKT.NZD 160/91 (1271.Z.21/4 September 1855), BOA A.MKT.NZD 235/31 (1274.M.14/4 September 1857), BOA A.MKT. NZD 241/78 (1274.Ra.26/14 November 1857), BOA Cevdet Belediye 93/4613 (19.N.1266/ 29 July 1850). See also Özbek, *Osmanlı İmparatorluğu'nda* on this issue.

45. BOA İ.MVL 91/1854 (1263.Ra.24/12 March 1847), BOA Cevdet Belediye 90/4467 (1255.Za.29/3 February 1840), BOA İ.MVL 112/2632 (1264.M.23/ 31 December 1847), BOA Cevdet Maliye 690/28280 (1267.Z.9/5 October 1851), BOA İ.MVL 228/7822 (1268.Ra.16/9 January 1852), BOA İ.MVL 263/997 (1269.Ca.22/3 March 1853), BOA İ.MVL 313/13122 (1270.Z.3), BOA İ.DH 295/18609 (1270.C.11/11 March 1854), BOA İ.MVL 391/17024 (1274.B.23/ 9 March 1858), BOA İ.MVL 408/17724 (1275.R.16/23 November 1858), BOA İ.MVL 397/17286 (1274.Za.23/5 July 1858), BOA İ.MVL 433/1910 (1276.Z.18/ 7 July1860), BOA A.MKT.MHM 191/99 (1277.M.27/15 August 1860), BOA DH.MKT 1594/28 (1306.C.12/13 February 1889), BOA DH.MKT 1772/33 (1308.Ra.2/16 October 1890), BOA DH.MKT 1913/16 (1309.C.18/19 January 1892), BOA DH.MKT 1993/49 (1310.S.4/28 September 1892). See also Maksudyan, 'Hearing the Voiceless'.
46. BOA İ.DH 1185/92723 (1307.Za.12/30 June 1890).
47. One of the few comprehensive studies on this issue is Nadir Özbek. See especially Chapter 5 'The Sultan and his Welfare Institutions: Symbols of Modernity and Progress'. See also see Maksudyan, 'Hearing the Voiceless'.
48. BOA ŞD 2393/39 (1288.S.29/20 May 1871).
49. BOA ZB 303/56 (1316.Kanunsani.3/16 January 1901), BOA ZB 301/14 (1317. Mart.04/17 March 190).
50. BOA İ.DH 1214/95051 (1308.Ca.10/22 December 1890).
51. BOA İ.DH 1214/95051 (1308.Ca.10/22 December 1890).
52. BOA İ.DH 1214/95051 (1308.Ca.10/22 December 1890). Although previously the wages were to be paid from the municipal budget, this document reports that funds from the budget of the Agricultural Bank could be allocated for this purpose. It is also important to note that although similar financial aid had previously been offered, it had only been given to families with more than seven children. The decision to reduce the number of children from seven to four as the precondition for aid also shows that the remedies were getting more practical and more effective.
53. BOA DH.MKT 1501/34 (1305.Ş.5/17 April 1888).
54. BOA DH.MKT 1481/55 (1305.Ca.16/30 January 1888).
55. Recently the evaluation of the Abdülhamid era has profoundly changed. Whereas previously scholars predominantly emphasized the oppressive aspects of the Abdülhamid era and argued that it was a period of hiatus in terms of modernization and a turning back to Islamic values, the recent scholarship has compellingly demonstrated that the increasing use of Islamic signs and symbols during this period was the very path of state modernization in the Ottoman context. For an approach that does an in-depth analysis of the means of sultanic legitimation see S. Deringil, *The Well-Protected Domains: Ideology and the Legitimation of Power in the Ottoman Empire, 1876–1909* (I. B. Tauris, 1999). For a subtle analysis of the formation of the welfare state and philantrophic activities in this period see Özbek, *Osmanlı İmparatorluğu'nda*; N. Ozbek, 'Philanthropic Activity, Ottoman Patriotism and the Hamidian Regime, 1876–1909', *International Journal of Middle East Studies,* 37:1 (2005), pp. 59–81; N. Ozbek, 'Imperial Gifts and Sultanic Legitimation During the Reign of Sultan Abdülhamid II, 1876–1909', in M. Ener, A. Singer and M. Bonner (eds), *Poverty and Charity in the Middle Eastern Con-*

texts (New York: University of New York Press, 2003). For a conceptual evaluation of the change of the scholarship see N. Özbek, 'Modernite, tarih ve İdeoloji: II. Abdülhamit Dönemi Tarihçiliği Üzerine bir Değerlendirme', *Türkiye Araştırmaları Literatür Dergisi*, 2:1 (2004), pp. 71–90; S. Deringil, 'New Approaches to the Study of the Ottoman Nineteenth Century', in Ç. Kafesçioğlu and L. Thys-Şenocak (eds), *Aptullah Kuran için Yazılar* (Istanbul: YKY, 1999); G. Çetinsaya, 'Abdülhamit'i Anlamak: 19. Yüzyıl Tarihçiliğine Bir Bakış', in K. Şahin, S. Sökmen and T. Bora (eds), *Sosyal Bilimleri Yeniden Düşünmek: Yeni bir Kavrayışa Doğru* (Istanbul: Metis, 1998), pp. 137–46.

56. BOA İ.DH 1185/92723 (1307.Za.12/30 June 1890).
57. BOA İ.DH 1185/92723 (1307.Za.12/30 June 1890).
58. BOA İ.DH 1185/92723 (1307.Za.12/30 June 1890). See also BOA MV 60/35 (1308. Ca.5/17 December 1890) for the Board of Ministers' (*Meclis-i Vükela*) follow-up meeting on this issue.
59. BOA Y.A.RES 61/15 (1310.Ra.14/6 October 1892).
60. BOA Y.A.RES 61/15 (1310.Ra.14/6 October 1892), Annex 2.
61. BOA Y.A.RES 61/15 (1310.Ra.14/6 October 1892), Annex 6.
62. BOA Y.A.RES 61/15 (1310.Ra.14/6 October 1892).
63. BOA Y.A.RES 61/15 (1310.Ra.14/6 October 1892).
64. H. Be. Paşa, *Iskat-ı Cenin: Facia* (Istanbul, 1290 (1873)).
65. Ibid., pp. 99–100.
66. 'Iskat-ı Cenin Yani Çocuk Düşürmek', *Ayine* (13 Z. 1292 (11 December 1975)), pp. 1–2. For information about the journal, *Ayine*, see A. Bozkurt, '93 Harbi Eşiğinde Selanik'te Bir Kadın Dergisi: Ayine (1875–1876)', *Kebikeç*, 19 (2005), pp. 73–97.
67. 'Iskat-ı Cenin Yani Çocuk Düşürmek'.
68. Ibid.
69. Ibid.
70. A. Rasim, 'Cenin' in *Servet-i Fünun*, 1:11 (1297), p. 125.
71. Ibid.
72. Ibid.
73. Ibid.
74. See for example, Namık Kemal, 'Iskat-ı Cenin', *Hadika*, 15 (27.N.1289/28 November 1872), and 'Nüfus', *İbret*, 9 (19R.1289/26 June 1872).
75. Namık Kemal, 'Iskat-ı Cenin', *Hadika*, 15 (27.N.1289/28 November 1872).
76. *Mecmua-i Fünun* was a major journal on science published by the Ottoman Society of Science (*Cemiyet-i İlmiye-i Osmaniye*) from 1862 until 1883. It was one of the main advocates of positivism in Ottoman society. The articles of the Ottoman men of science presenting the contemporary scientific approaches and developments were published in the journal. These articles ranged from physics, chemistry, jeology, and medicine to history, geography, philosophy and logic. For *Mecmua-i Fünun*, see Y. Işıl, 'Bir Aydınlanma Hareketi Olarak Mecmua-i Fünun' (MA Thesis, İstanbul University, 1986), C. Aydın, 'Mecmua-i Fünun ve Mecmua-i Ulum Dergilerinin Medeniyet ve Bilim Anlayışı' (MA Thesis, Istanbul University, 1995). Y. I. Ülman, 'Mecmua-i Fünûn'da Tıp Konulu Yazılar', *Bilim Tarihi*, 22 (1993), pp. 17–30.
77. Aziz, 'Iskat-ı Cenin', *Mecmua-i Fünun*, 41 (December 1866), pp. 289–92. Demirci and Somel, 'Women's Bodies' also present and analyse the anti-abortion discourses in detail.
78. M. Süreyya, 'Kırımlızade Aziz İdris', in *Sicill-i Osmani*, 6 vols (Istanbul: Kültür Bakanlığı ve Türkiye Ekonomik ve Toplumsal Tarih Vakfı, 1996), vol. 2, p. 345.
79. Aziz, 'Iskat-ı Cenin'.

80. Abortion was harmful in two ways: the first was for the individual and the second was for the public, according to Aziz's framework. The individual harms were harms given to the body. In order to force an expulsion of the foetus, women swallowed sabin, rue, and ergot of rye (*Lolium temulentum*), drew blood, had somebody bluntly hit her belly, or killed the fetus by inserting something into the womb. It is obvious that such methods would affect and kill the mother before she dropped her baby. When it came to public harm, abortion would lead to depopulation, and eventually hamper the progress and happiness of the country.
81. Aziz, 'Iskat-ı Cenin'.
82. Ibid.
83. BOA İ.DH 1185/92723 (1307.Za.12/30 June 1890).
84. See Demirci and Somel, 'Women's Bodies', for an analysis of the representations of abortion in advice literature and the press.
85. Ibid.
86. H. Be. Paşa, *Iskat-ı Cenin. Facia* (Istanbul: 13 No.lu Matbaa, 1290 (1874–5)).
87. This novel has first been censured when it was being published in a newspaper in episodes and has never been published in Ottoman Turkish. Today it is possible to find its transcribed reprints. See Uşaklıgil, Halid Ziya, Sefile (Istanbul: Özgür Yayınları, 2006).
88. Karpat, *Ottoman Population*.

4 Pregnancy as a Site of Medical Intervention

1. For example, see Abdülaziz Bey, *Osmanlı Adet, Merasim*. Balıkhane Nazırı Ali Rıza Bey, *Bir Zamanlar İstanbul* (Tercüman 1001 Temel Eser); K. Arısan, 'Doğum Yardımının Dünü, Bugünü ve Bizde Ev-Saray Doğumlarıyla İlgili Gelenekler', *İstanbul Üniversitesi Tıp Fakültesi Mecmuası*, 43:85 (1980); K. Arısan, 'Geçen Yüzyılda İstanbul'da Ebeler ve Doğum', in *1. Türk Tıp Tarihi Kongresi, İstanbul 17–19 Şubat 1988, Bildiriler* (Ankara: 1992), pp. 253–59; M. Cemiloğlu, *Halk Hikayelerinde Doğum Motifi* (Bursa: Uludağ Üniversitesi Güçlendirme Vakfı, 1999); O. Acıpayamlı, *Türkiyede Doğumla İlgili Adet ve İnanmaların Etnolojik Etüdü* (1961); A. S. Unver, 'Tarihte Ebeler ve Doğum Tarihimiz', in *II. Ana Sağlığı Semineri* (Istanbul: 1967). It is also interesting that popular believes on childbed fever, which was known as *albastı*, have received considerable attention. See for example, E. Simsek, 'Çukurova'da Anlatılan 'Alkarısı' Efsanelerinin Türk Efsaneleri İçindeki Yeri', in *I. Uluslararası Karacaoğlan ve Çukurova Halk Kültürü Sempozyumu* (21–3 Kasım 1990, Adana) *Bildiriler* (Adana, 1991); İ. Z. Eyüboğlu, *Anadolu İnançları Anadolu Mitologisi:İnanç-Söylence Bağlantısı* (Istanbul: Geçit Kitabevi, 1987); M Y. Helimoğlu, *Diyarbakır Efsaneleri; Derleme-Araştırma-İnceleme* (Ankara: Doruk, 1993); N. Elmacı, 'Doğum Gelenekleri: Bakacak Köyünün Dünü ve Bugünu', *Folklor Edebiyat*, 30:2 (2002), pp. 329–46.
2. M. K. Matossian, and S. Hoogasian Villa, *1914 Öncesi Ermeni Köy Hayatı*, trans. Altuğ Yılmaz (Istanbul: Aras Yayıncılık, 2006).
3. C. Delaney, C., *The Seed and the Soil: Gender and Cosmology in Turkish Village* (Berkeley, CA: University of California, 1991).
4. L. A. Pollock, 'Embarking on a Rough Passage: The Experience of Maternity in Early Modern Society', in D. McLaren and V. A. Fildes (eds), *Women as Mothers in Pre-industrial England: Essays in Memory of Dorothy McLaren* (London: Routledge, 1990), pp. 39–67.
5. Broomhall, 'Women's Little Secrets', pp. 1–15.

6. U. Rublack, 'Pregnancy, Childbirth and the Female Body in Early Modern Germany', *Past and Present*, 150 (1996), pp. 84–110.
7. M. H. Green, 'From "Diseases of Women" to "Secrets of Women": The Transformation of Gynecological Literature in the Later Middle Ages', *Journal of Medieval and Early Modern Studies*, 30:1 (2000), pp. 5–39.
8. L. Tatlock, 'Speculum Feminarum: Gendered Perspectives on Obstetrics and Gynecology in Early Modern Germany', *Signs*, 17:4 (1992), pp. 725–60.
9. R. Kukla, *Mass Hysteria: Medicine, Culture, and Mothers' Bodies* (London: Rowman and Littlefield, 2005).
10. B. Duden, *The Woman Beneath the Skin: A Doctor's Patients in Eighteenth-Century Germany* (Boston, MA: Harvard University Press, 1991); also see B. Duden, *Disembodying Women: Perspectives on Pregnancy and the Unborn*, trans. Lee Hoinacki (Cambridge, MA: Harvard University Press, 1993).
11. Kukla, *Mass Hysteria*.
12. Skanzoni, *Fenn-i Vilade*.
13. Halid Ziya (Uşaklıgil), *Haml-ü Vaz'ı Haml* (Istanbul: Mihran Matbaası, 1306 (1888/9)).
14. A. Debay, *Hygiène et physiologie du mariage; histoire naturelle et médicale de l'homme et de la femme mariés; dans ses plus curieux détails. Théorie nouvelle de la procréation mâle et femelle, stérilité, impuissance, imperfections génitales, moyens de les combattre. Hygiène spéciale de la femme enceinte et du nouveau-né* (Paris: E. Dentu, 1859).
15. Besim Ömer, *Gebelik ve Gebelikte Tedabir* (Istanbul, 1318 (1900/1)).
16. Besim Ömer had also produced medical treatises written for the students of medicine and midwifery training, as well as advice books for midwives that described the process of gestation, the mechanics of parturition and the possible complications in the pre- and post-natal periods. Again despite the lack of information regarding the number of copies printed and sold, the availability of different editions suggest that his books have been widely read. His five-volume book *Fenn-i Velade* was a medical treatise to be used in obstetrics courses. *Ebelik* was also a medical treatise to be used in midwifery courses. *Ebe Hanımlara Öğütlerim* was a prescriptive manual that mainly set the moral standards for the midwives. However, it also included a brief discussion of the process and mechanics of parturition. *Ebelik, Doğurmak ve Doğurtmak*, on the other hand, can be called a medical treatise for midwives by its scope and tone. This book opens with a reprint of the former manual but after that, it presents an elaborate and scholarly discussion about the process of gestation, the mechanics of childbirth, and pre- and post-natal medical care, which is comparable to those in the books for medical students. See Besim Ömer, *Fenn-i Velade* (Istanbul: Ahmet İhsan Matbaası, 1933); Besim Ömer, *Ebelik* (Istanbul: Ahmet İhsan Matbaası, 1928); Ömer, *Ebe Hanımlara Öğütlerim*; Ömer, *Ebelik, Doğurmak ve Doğurtmak*.
17. 'Gebelik ve Gebelikte Tedabir', in *Servet-i Fünun*, 24:615 (23 November 1318/5 February 1903), pp. 208–9.
18. Although Debay's work was a bestselling book on sexuality, Halid Ziya had selectively chosen the parts about pregnancy and excluded the gist of the book. This of course deserves a separate discussion on its own account.
19. 'Disciplining women in a good way is equal to disciplining the children, the grand children, and hence the humankind itself. The health, physical constitution, and character of the children are dependent upon the mother's health, and bound to the precautions and corroborations of the mother to maintain hygiene both for herself and for her children.' Besim Ömer, *Gebelik ve Gebelikte Tedabir*, p. 1.

20. For example: 'All the topics and talks about the discipline of female body and female mind deserve attention and are essential for the peace and profit of humankind. A woman is the field where human kind grows on and feeds upon. A woman complements the man and she is the garden of humanity. Therefore, the effort spent for the bodily and moral discipline of women is the most admired of all the service for civilization, the most sacred of all human duty, and deserves attention and appreciation the most of all work for social and moral progress.' Besim Ömer, *Gebelik ve Gebelikte Tedabir*, p. 1.
21. 'Family means woman; the happiness of the family depends on the investment on and discipline of woman.' Besim Ömer, *Gebelik ve Gebelikte Tedabir*, p. 7.
22. 'Spending effort for the bodily and moral discipline of a young girl is helping the formation of a good mother because that bodily and moral discipline would not be reserved only for that girl but would pass on to her children due to her motherhood. There is no doubt that the whole family would benefit from the influencing felicity signs of this admired physical and moral situation.' Besim Ömer, *Gebelik ve Gebelikte Tedabir*, p. 2.
23. 'The children and the grand children should first be disciplined bodily and morally before anything else, since moral discipline is only possible through the completion and complacency of the bodily discipline.' Besim Ömer, *Gebelik ve Gebelikte Tedabir*, p. 2.
24. 'Being deprived of motherhood is like pus dripping drop by drop from the poisoned place. One feels it as if God had placed an empty cradle that cannot bear being empty to the lap of women'. Besim Ömer, *Gebelik ve Gebelikte Tedabir*, p. 1.
25. Ibid., p. 42.
26. Ibid., p. 15. I want to remind readers that it was strictly forbidden for midwives to turn the baby inside the uterus. Moreover, use of forceps was a prerogative of the physicians. See Chapter 2 of this work.
27. Similar ideas are also expressed in Besim Ömer, *Gebe Hanımlara Öğütlerim*.
28. Halid Ziya (Uşaklıgil), *Haml-ü Vaz'-ı Haml*, p. 28.
29. See also L. Schiebinger, *Nature's Body: Gender in the Making of Modern Science* (Boston, MA: Beacon Press, 1993).
30. Besim Ömer, *Gebelik ve Gebelikte Tedabir*, pp. 114–16.
31. Ibid., p. 91.
32. Ibid., p. 92.
33. 'One of the primary rights of children is to be born in a good shape.' Ibid., p. 93.
34. 'The mothers should avoid sexual intercourse during pregnancy to protect the health and wellbeing of her child. The first step on the road to human culture is the control of appetite. Those who cannot consent and follow a moderate lifestyle for the benefit of their unborn children have to give up fatherhood. (taken from Alis Istokham).' Ibid., *Gebelik ve Gebelikte Tedabir*, p. 93.
35. 'Although all mothers wish their children to have beauty and well constitution, the accomplishment of this wish is possible only through full concordance with the rules of hygiene. It is natural that the newborns of those mothers who do not take the necessary precautions and ignore to change their lifestyles during pregnancy would have some deficiencies.' Halid Ziya (Uşaklıgil), *Haml-ü Vaz'ı Haml*, p. 17.
36. 'A mother who finds out that a body is developing within her own body should adapt her lifestyle and routines to the needs of the new one, and should change her behaviour for the baby's serenity and health.' Ibid., p. 4.
37. 'The human need for hygiene dates back to the emergence to life. Because of this, the parents are responsible to care and take the precautions for the health of their child who is incapable of satisfying her own needs yet.' Ibid., p. 4.

38. 'The tasks and duty of motherhood starts when one realizes pregnancy. The pregnant woman should devote all of her action to the body that she carries and she should devoid herself of all her feminine pleasures and interests as well as villainous acts that would bring harms later. That way, the newborn would acquire decorations that are naturally wished for, such as beauty, strength, and health.' Ibid., pp. 7–8.
39. Ibid., pp. 66–9.
40. 'Those who want to avoid that grave danger (death) should behave in conformity with the list provided above and with consideration of the knowledge about hygiene that we discussed previously. Otherwise, those mothers who are expecting the fruit of their life would end up having nothing but a lifeless corpse.' Ibid., p.70.
41. 'Since pregnant women become very fragile and emotional toward the end of pregnancy, one should approach them very carefully and sensitively. Because they become extremely tender and sore from the slightest events, their health becomes more erratic than usual in the final stages of pregnancy. One should deal with a pregnant woman as if she is a child, tell her amusing stories and interesting jokes, and try to overcome the gloominess of their conscience'. Ibid., p. 63.
42. Ibid., pp. 43–53.
43. Ibid., p. 65.
44. Halid Ziya (Uşaklıgil), *Kanun ve Fenn-i Vilade* (Istanbul: Nişan Berberyan Matbaası, 1311 (1893)).
45. Debay, *Hygiène et physiologie du mariage,* p.
46. Halid Ziya (Uşaklıgil), *Kanun ve Fenn-i Vilade*, p. 9.
47. Ibid.
48. Ibid., p. 10.
49. Ibid., pp. 10–11.
50. Ibid., p. 26.
51. Ibid., p. 27.
52. Ibid., p. 28.
53. Ibid., p. 32.
54. Ibid., p. 36.
55. Ibid., p. 38.
56. 'The precautions to secure the facial beauty and the proportion of the body depend, first of all, on the discipline and the duties fulfilled by the mother.' Ibid., p. 66
57. Ibid., p. 39.
58. Ibid., p. 30.
59. Ibid., p. 31.
60. Ibid., p. 29.
61. H. Aynur, 'Malumatçı Baba Tahir', 'Baba Tahir, [Publisher] of Malumat', *Toplumsal Tarih*, 128 (2004), pp. 62–5.
62. For a critical approach to Seyyid Tahir, see I. C. Schick, 'Print Capitalism and Women's Sexual Agency in the Late Ottoman Empire', *Comparative Studies of South Asia, Africa and the Middle East*, 31:1 (2011), pp. 196–216.
63. For a subtle analysis of the context within which the journals for women emerged, see Schick, 'Print Capitalism and Women's Sexual Agency'. See also T. Demirci, 'Body, Disease and Late Ottoman Literature: Debates on Ottoman Muslim Family in the Tanzimat Period (1839–1908)' (PhD Dissertation, Bilkent University, 2008); Aprahamian and Rowe (eds), *Ottoman Women's Movements and Print Cultures.*
64. S. Tahir, *Vaz'ı Haml: İbtia-ı Hamil, Kabilenin Vazifesi, Cenin* (Istanbul: Şems Matbaası, 1331 (1915), p. 3.

65. Ibid., p. 4.
66. Ibid., p. 4.
67. Ibid., pp. 6, 7.
68. S. G. Salgırlı, 'Eugenics as Science of the Social: A Case from 1930s Istanbul' (PhD Dissertation, Binghamton University, 2009).
69. Salgırlı, *Eugenics as Science of the Social.*
70. A. Debay, *Sıhhatnüma-yı İzdivac: Evleneceklerle Müteehhil ve Mücerred Bulunanlara Nasihat*, trans. Besim Ömer (Istanbul: Alem Matbaası, 1306 (1888/9)).
71. Besim Ömer, *Fen ve izdivac: Evlenebilecekler ve Evlenemeyecekler* (Istanbul: Yeni Matbaa, 1340 (1921/2)).
72. Seyyid Tahir, *Vaz'ı Haml*, p. 4.
73. Ibid., p. 5.
74. Ibid.
75. Ibid., p. 6.
76. Ibid., p. 6.
77. Girlhood as a historical category has remained almost totally unexamined in the Ottoman context with the exception of E. E. Akşit, 'Girls' Education and the Paradoxes of Modernity and Nationalism in the Late Ottoman Empire and the Early Turkish Republic' (PhD Dissertation, Binghamton University, 2004); and also E. E. Akşit, 'Rearrangement of the Public and the Private Spheres', in D. Köksal and A. Falierou (eds), *Ottoman Women: A Social History from 19th and 20th Centuries* (London: I. B. Tauris, forthcoming).
78. *Her Genç Kız Neler Bilmelidir?* (Istanbul: Sevimli Ay Matbaası, 1926).
79. For the political definition and uses of the girlhood in the Early Turkish Republic, see Akşit, *Girls'* and Akşit, 'Rearrangement of the Public and the Private Spheres'.
80. Seyyid Tahir, *Vaz'ı Haml*, pp. 9, 10.
81. Ibid., p. 11
82. Ibid., p. 14.

5 Infertility as a Public Problem

1. Besim Ömer, *Gebelik ve Gebelikte Tedabir*, p. 1.
2. See for example, *Hanım Kızlara* (Istanbul: A. Maviyan Şirket-i Mürettibiye Matbaası, 1304 (1887)); *Hanımlara Mahsus Malûmat* (Istanbul, 1895); Hüseyin Remzi, *Mir'atü'l-beyt. Hanımlara Yadigar* (İstanbul, 1891); Avanzade Mehmed Süleyman, *Gençlerde İstimna Bi-l-yed* (Istanbul: Kader Matbaası, 1329 (1913)).
3. Mustafa Safi, *Evlendirecek, Evlenecek ve Evlenmişlere Mahsus Saadet-i İzdivac* (Istanbul: Asır Matbaası, 1325 (1907/8); Avanzade Mehmed Süleyman, *Yeni, Mükemmel, Son Rehber-i İzdivac* (Istanbul: el-Adl Matbaası, 1338 (1922)). A. Naci, *Rehnüma-yı İzdivac* (Istanbul: Manzume-i Efkâr Matbaası, 1328 (1912)); Mustafa Safi, *Saadet-i İzdivac* (Istanbul: Asır Matbaası, 1325 (1907)); Hüseyin Remzi, *Sağdıç Rehber-i İzdivac* (Istanbul: Artin Asaduryan Şirket-i Mürettibiye Matbaası, 1315 (1899)); Necmeddin Sami, *Sevda Çiçekleri yahud İzdivacın Ehemmiyeti* (Istanbul: Kasbar Matbaası, 1312 (1895)); Ş. Ka (Talimcioğlu), *Hıfz-ı Sıhhat-i İzdivaç* (Istanbul: Kasbar Matbaası, 1310 (1893)): Ahmed Said, *Hıfz-ı Sıhhat-i İzdivaç ve Tenasül* (Istanbul: Kasbar Matbaası, 1308 (1891)); R. Hüseyin, *Müntehebat-ı Hüseyin Remzi'den Hayat Memat ve Aşk İzdivaç* (Istanbul: Artin Asaduryan Şirket-i Mürettebiye matbaası). In this period a periodical on marriage was also published. See *İzdivaç: İlmî, Edebî, İçtimai ve Sıhhi Musavver*

Mecmua (Istanbul, 1918). M. Faik, *Saadet-i Aile* (Istanbul: A. Asaduryan Şirket-i Mürettibiye Matbaası, 1316 (1899)). These books also took the family as the main unit, and directed their advice toward family relationships. See Besim Ömer, *Sıhhatnümâ-yı Aile yahud Baba, Ana, Çocuk* (Istanbul: Mahmud Bey Matbaası, 1304 (1887)); Hüseyin Remzi, *Yadigâr-ı Remzi: Aile Hıfzı's-sıhhası* (İstanbul: A. Asaduryan Şirket-i Mürettibiye Matbaası, 1900); H. Hamid, *Yeni Aile Rehberi* (Istanbul: Hukuk Matbaası, 1919); S. Saim [Unar], *Ana Baba Nasihatları* (Istanbul: Kasbar Matbaası, 1889); A. Midhat, *Ana Babanın Evlât Üzerindeki Hukuk ve Vazâifi* (Istanbul: Tercüman-ı Hakikat Matbaası, 1899). For an evaluation of advice literature in relation to the ideals of the family in the Tanzimat period, see Demirci *Body, Disease and Late Ottoman Literature: Debates on Ottoman Muslim Family in the Tanzimat Period (1839–1908)*.

4. A. Debay, *Sıhhatnüma-yı İzdivac: Evleneceklerle Müteehhil ve Mücerred Bulunanlara Nasihat*, trans. Besim Ömer (İstanbul: Alem Matbaası, 1306 (1888/9)); Besim Ömer, *Fen ve izdivac: Evlenebilecekler ve Evlenemeyecekler* (Istanbul: Yeni Matbaa, 1340 (1921/2)).
5. Avanzade Mehmed Süleyman (trans.), *Kız mı oğlan mı?* (Is it a Girl or a Boy?) (Dersaadet (Istanbul): Araks Matbaası, 1330 (1914)), for a later book see *Kız mı oğlan mı?* (Istanbul: Sevimli Ay Matbaası, 1927).
6. S. Çakır, *Osmanlı Kadın Hareketi* (Istanbul: Metis Yayınları, 1994), A. Demirdirek, *Osmanlı Kadınlarının Hayat Hakkı Arayışının Bir Hikayesi* (Ankara: İmge Kitabevi, 1993); A. İlyasoğlu and D. İnsel, 'Kadın Dergilerinin Evrimi', in *Türkiye'de Dergiler, Ansiklopediler (1849–1984)* (Istanbul: Gelişim Yayınları, 1984), pp. 163–83; V. D. Altınöz, 'The Ottoman Women's Movement: Women's Press, Magazines, Journals, and Newspapers from 1875 to 1923' (MA thesis, University of Miami, 2003); A. Karakaya-Stump, 'Debating Progress in a "Serious Newspaper for Muslim Women": The Periodical Kadın of the Post-revolutionary Salonica, 1908–1909', *British Journal of Middle Eastern Studies*, 30:2 (2003), pp. 155–81; Y. Akpolat, *Sosyoloji Araştırmaları: Osmanlı'da Kadın Dergileri ve Sosyoloji Dergileri* (Istanbul: Fenomen Yayıncılık, 2004); F. Kılıç, 'Kadın: A Young Turk Magazine in the Second Constitutional Period (1908–1909)' (MA thesis, Boğaziçi University, 2005); F. Kılıç Denman, *İkinci Meşrutiyet Döneminde bir Jön Türk Dergisi: 'Kadın'* (A Young Turk Magazine in the Second Constitutional Period: Kadın) (Istanbul: Libra Yayıncılık, 2010); for a critical evolution of the secondary literature and an analysis of the political context within which the periodicals for women emerged, see Schick, 'Print Capitalism and Women's Sexual Agency', pp. 196–216.
7. S. Tosunpaşazade, *Muamelat-ı Zevciyede Adem-i İktidar* (Istanbul: Şems Matbaası, 1328/30 (1912)); Avanzade Mehmed Süleyman, *Yalnız Erkeklere Mahsus Adem-i İktidar* (Istanbul: Kasbar Matbaası, 1330/2 (1914)).
8. Besim Ömer, *Ukm ve Ananet* (Dersaâdet: Mahmud Bey Matbaası, 1306 (1890–1)), p. 13. The name of this book is catalogued wrongly as 'Ukm ve İnanet' in most of the library collections when transcribed from Arabic script to Latin script. In Ottoman Turkish, there is no word as 'inanet' but 'ananet', which is impotence. Here I will use the correct transcription.
9. Ibid., p. 12.
10. Ibid., p. 10.
11. Ibid., p. 5.
12. Besim Ömer, *Gebelik ve Gebelikte Tedabir*, p. 1.
13. Besim Ömer, *Ukum ve Ananet*, pp. 22–35.
14. Ibid., p. 22.

15. Ibid., p. 38.
16. 'The example that 'all trees that flower will also naturally yield fruits in the end' is not so correct.' Ibid., p. 73.
17. 'Although some old trees in our gardens still flower and herald the coming of the spring with their fragrances, the slightest wind and withers and stripes them of their flowers. Indeed, such flowers are the 'farewell' kisses of those old trees.' Ibid., p. 74.
18. On this issue, see Ornella Moscucci, *The Science of Woman*.
19. I borrow this usage in the specific context of infertility from A. L. Greil, 'Infertile Bodies: Medicalization, Metaphor, and Agency', in M. Inhorn and F. Van Balen (eds) *Infertility Around the Globe* (Berkeley, CA: University of California Press, 2002), pp. 101–19, on p. 102.
20. For a discussion of the roles of local midwifes and folk practices in curing infertility in Turkey, see F. Gökçen Dinç, 'Ignorant, Dirty, Superstitious Crones: Degrading of Midwifery and Midwives in Modern Turkey' (MA Thesis, Istanbul Bilgi University, 2011).
21. Besim Ömer, *Ukum ve Ananet*, p. 50.
22. Ibid., pp. 50–4.
23. Ibid., p. 72.
24. 'To a woman whose uterus is a bended forward: 'Please do not go to the toilet and urinate for five or six hours before the sexual intercourse on the evenings that you are likely to get involved. Do not get anxious by imagining how that would work. That is not your business. All you have to do is to avoid urinating. After the sexual intercourse you can urinate, not before'.
    'To a woman whose uterus is a bended backward: Toward the termination of your menstruation, eat lots of eggs and rice. You will also need to swallow those small pills that I prepare, three or four times in the evenings. All those pills contain is two and half centigrams of opium extraction each. You would prepare yourself not to go to the toilet for three or four days. You will first have sexual intercourse and then go to the toilet'.
    The prominent German doctor and writer named Hanri Kiş, in his book 'Female Infertility' that was published this year, advises couples to get involved in sexual intercourse in a position where the woman is on top of her husband in the cases of retroversion or when part of her vagina is bended forward. According to him in that position, the mouth of the uterus will fall downward and forward while part of the vagina will move backward'. Ibid., pp. 67–70.
25. Avanzade Mehmed Süleyman, *Mesail-i Mühimme-i Hayatiye ve Sıhhiyeden Kısır Kadınlar* (Istanbul: Kader Matbaası, 1336 (1920)).
26. Mehmet Süleyman (Avanzade) was born in 1871. He was trained in pharmacy at the School of Medicine. While he was working as a pharmacist, he started writing on contemporary issues. He wrote and published many books, and he published several best selling journals including Afiyet and Güzel Prenses (Beautiful Princess). His interests covered many different topics such as crime fiction, culinary books, popular history works, and popular medicine works. Most of all, he was the publisher of first women's year book, *Nevsal-i Nisvan*. See *Tanzimat'tan Bugüne Edebiyatçılar Ansiklopedisi*, 2 vols (Istanbul: YKY, 2001), vol. 2, p. 558.
27. Avanzade Mehmed Süleyman, *Yalnız Erkeklere Mahsus Adem-i İktidar*.
28. 'Although infertility protects the beauty of the body, it is a quality that does not have any benefits at all for the human society.' Ibid., cover.
29. Halid Ziya (Uşaklıgil), *Kanun ve Fenn-i Vilade*.
30. Ibid.

31. 'Infertile woman is like a tree the fruit of which is inedible. Both should be grafted and ameliorated.'. Avanzade Mehmed Süleyman *Kısır Kadınlar*, cover, see also pp. 7, 9, 15.
32. Ibid., p. 4.
33. Ibid.
34. Ibid.
35. Besim Ömer, *Ukm ve Ananet.*
36. Avanzade Mehmed Süleyman, *Kısır Kadınlar*, p. 7.
37. Ibid., p. 20.
38. Ibid., p. 21.
39. Ibid., p. 15.
40. Besim Ömer, *Ukum ve Ananet*, pp. 121–4.
41. Ibid., p. 10.
42. Avanzade Mehmed Süleyman, *Kısır Kadınlar*, p. 5.
43. 'Both for women and men, as the genitals become better the fertility increase.' Debay, *Sıhhatnüma-yı İzdivac*, pp. 82–5. Although this book was not written but translated by Besim Ömer, I will discuss it as representative of Besim Ömer's ideas on infertility.
44. N. Fuad, *İzdivac: Şerait-i Sıhhiye ve İctimaiyesi* (Dersaadet: Orhaniye Matbaası, 1342 (1923)), p. 35.
45. Ibid., p. 69.
46. Ibid.
47. Ibid. Hüseyin Remzi, *Sağdıç-Rehber-i İzdivaç* (Istanbul: A.[rtin] Asaduryan Şirket-i Mürettibiye Matbaası, 1315 (1897)). Avanzade Mehmed Süleyman, *Yeni, Mükemmel, Son Rehber-i İzdivac* (Istanbul: el-Adl Matbaası, 1338 (1922)).
48. See also the books on impotence. S. Tosunpaşazade, *Muamelat-ı Zevciyede Adem-i İktidar*; Avanzade Mehmed Süleyman, *Yalnız Erkeklere Mahsus Adem-i İktidar*; Halid Ziya (Uşaklıgil), *Kanun ve Fenn-i Vilade.*
49. Avanzade Mehmed Süleyman, *Kısır Kadınlar*, p. 24.
50. In many of his works, it is possible to find this stereotyping as I discussed in Chapter 1 of this work. See for example, Besim Ömer, *Doğum Tarihi* (Istanbul: Ahmed İhsan Matbaası, 1932); Besim Ömer, *Ebe Hanımlara Öğütlerim*; Besim Ömer, *Ebelik, Doğurmak ve Doğurtmak*; Besim Ömer *Ebelik.*
51. Besim Ömer, *Ukum ve Ananet*, pp. 87–8.
52. Ibid., pp. 86–9.
53. Fuad, *İzdivac*, p. 36, and Hüseyin Remzi, *Sağdıç-Rehber-i İzdivaç.*
54. Besim Ömer, *Ukum ve Ananet*, p. 92.
55. Avanzade Mehmed Süleyman, *Kısır Kadınlar*, p. 24.
56. Besim Ömer, *Fenn-ü İzdivac*, pp. 76–7. See the part titled, 'Marriage and Children'.
57. The books on impotence also emphasize this point.
58. Avanzade Mehmed Süleyman, *Kısır Kadınlar*, p. 24.
59. Hüseyin Remzi, *Sağdıç-Rehber-i İzdivaç*, p. 65
60. Ibid., pp. 68–70.
61. Fuad, *İzdivac*, p. 69.
62. 'If a woman does not get married until she is thirty five or forty she would not be able to conceive since she would lose her ability to give birth almost totally for not being used for long years.' Fuad, *İzdivac*, p. 70.
63. The literature on impotence again includes very detailed descriptions of these methods.
64. Debay, *Sıhhatnüma-yı İzdivac*, p. 83.
65. Besim Ömer, *Ukum ve Ananet*, pp. 15–18

66. Besim Ömer, *Ukum ve Ananet*, p. 19.
67. Ibid., p. 16.
68. Halid Ziya (Uşaklıgil), *Kanun ve Fenn-i Vilade*, p. 25.
69. Ibid., pp. 24–5.
70. Besim Ömer, *Kanun ve Fenn-i Vilade*, pp. 26–8.
71. Debay, *Sıhhatnüma-yı İzdivac*, pp. 82–3.
72. Fuad, *İzdivac*, p. 70.
73. Besim Ömer, *Ukum ve Ananet*, p. 78.
74. Ibid., p. 78.
75. Fuad, *İzdivac*, p. 83; Debay, *Sıhhatnüma-yı İzdivac*, pp. 215–24.
76. Halid Ziya (Uşaklıgil), *Kanun ve Fenn-i Vilade*, p. 46.
77. Ibid., p. 48.
78. Ibid., p. 49
79. Ibid., pp. 49–50.
80. Ibid., pp. 46–7.
81. Ibid., pp. 50–3.
82. Ibid., p. 53.
83. Ibid., pp. 53–4.
84. Ibid., p. 54
85. Ibid., pp. 54–61.
86. Ibid., p. 62.
87. Besim Ömer, *Fenn-ü İzdivac*, pp. 76–7. See the part titled 'Marriage and Children'.
88. Besim Ömer, *Fenn-ü İzdivac*, p. 77.
89. Ibid., p. 77.
90. Avanzade Mehmed Süleyman, *Kısır Kadınlar*, p. 16.
91. Ibid., p. 17.
92. *Gebe Kalmamak İçin Ne Yapmalı*? (Istanbul: Sevimli Ay Matbaası, 1927).

WORKS CITED

Archival Sources

Prime Ministry Archives (BOA-Başbakanlık Osmanlı Arşivi)

Classifications (Tasnifler) with individual documents

Cevdet Dahiliye.

Cevdet Sıhhiye.

A.DVN (Sadaret Divan Kalemi Evrakı).

A.DVN.MKT (Sadaret Divan Kalemi Evrakı Mektubi Kalemi).

A.MKT (Sadaret Mektubi Kalemi Evrakı).

A.MKT.MVL (Sadaret Meclis-i Vala Evrakı).

A.MKT.NZD (Sadaret Nezaret ve Devair Evrakı).

A.MKT.UM (Sadaret Umum Vilayat Evrakı).

DH.MKT (Dahiliye Nezareti Mektubi Kalemi).

HAT (Hatt-ı Hümayun).

HR.TO (Hariciye Nezareti Tercüme Odası).

İ.DH (İrade Dahiliye).

İ.HUS (İrade Hususi).

İ.MVL (İrade Meclis-i Vala).

İ.ŞD (İrade Şura-yı Devlet).

MF.ALY (Maarif Nezareti Mekatib-i Aliye).

MF.İST (Maarif Nezareti İstatistik Kalemi).

MF.VRK (Maarif Nezareti Evrak Odası).

MV (Meclis-i Vükela Mazbataları).

ŞD.Dersaadet (Şura-yı Devlet Dersaadet).

ŞD.Maarif (Şura-yı Devlet Maarif).

ZB (Zaptiye Nezareti).

Registers (Defterler)

Ayniyat Defterleri.

NGG Sıhhiye Gelen-Giden.

NGG Tıbbiye Gelen-Giden.

Court Registers

Burhaniye 1101, 1103.

Edremit 1259, 1260, 1261.

Besim Ömer's Books

Sıhhatnümâ-yı Aile yahud Baba, Ana, Çocuk (The Ways for the Health of the Family or of the Father, Mother, and Child) (Istanbul: Mahmud Bey Matbaası, 1304 (1886/7)).

Gebelik ve Gebelikte Tedabir (Pregnancy and the Precautions during Pregnancy) (Istanbul, 1318 (1900/1)).

Ebe Hanımlara Öğütlerim (My Advice to the Midwives) (Istanbul: Ahmed İhsan Matbaası, 1322 (1904/5)).

Ebelik, Doğurmak ve Doğurtmak (Midwifery, to Give Birth and to Deliver) (Istanbul: Ahmet İhsan Matbaası, 1322 (1904/5)).

Ukm ve Ananet (Infertility and Impotence) (Dersaâdet: Mahmud Bey Matbaası, 1306 (1890/1)).

Fenn-i Vilade (The Science of Birth) (Istanbul: Ahmet İhsan Matbaası, 1338 (1919/20)).

Ebelik (Midwifery) (Istanbul: Ahmet İhsan Matbaası, 1928).

Fen ve izdivac: Evlenebilecekler ve Evlenemeyecekler (Science and Marriage: Those Who Could and Could Not Get Married) (Istanbul: Yeni Matbaa, 1340 (1921/2)).

Doğum Tarihi (The History of Childbirth) (Istanbul: Ahmed İhsan Matbaası, 1932).

'Ebelik ve Doğum: Bizde Nasıldı ve Ne Haldedir?' (Midwifery and Childbirth: How was it Used to Be an How is It Right Now in Our Country), in *Sıhhat Almanağı* (The Yearbook of Health), ed. Mazhar Osman (Istanbul: Kader Matbaası, 1933).

Türk Çocuğunu Nasıl Yaşatmalı? (How Are We Going the Keep the Turkish Child Alive?) (Istanbul: Ahmed Ihsan Basımevi, 1939).

Published Sources

'50 Yıllık Ebe Sahin Anlatiyor!' (Fifty Years of Experienced Midwife Sahin Tells!), *Yeni İnci*, 11:32 (1953), pp. 10–12, p. 16.

'Gebelik ve Gebelikte Tedabir' (Pregnancy and Precautions during Pregnancy), *Servet-i Fünun*, 24:615 (23 November 1318/5 February 1903), pp. 208–9.

'İki Ebe Bir Gebe' (Two Midwives and One Pregnant), *Hayâl-i Cedîd*, 55–60 (28 October 1910–18 November 1910).

'Iskat-ı Cenin Yani Çocuk Düşürmek' (Dropping a Foetus or Abortion), in *Ayine* (13 Z. 1292 (11 December 1875)), pp. 1–2.

Ahmed Midhat, *Ana Babanın Evlât Üzerindeki Hukuk ve Vazâifi* (The Rights and the Duties of the Mother and Father on the Child) (Istanbul: Tercüman-ı Hakikat Matbaası, 1899).

Ahmed Naci, *Rehnüma-yı İzdivac* (Marriage Guide) (Istanbul: Manzume-i Efkâr Matbaası, 1328 (1910/11)).

Ahmed Said, *Hıfz-ı Sıhhat-i İzdivaç ve Tenasül* (The Hygiene of Marriage and Reproduction) (Istanbul: Kasbar Matbaası, 1308 (1890/1)).

Ahmet Rasim, 'Cenin' (Foetus), *Servet-i Fünun*, 1:11 (1297), p. 125.

Avanzade M. Süleyman, *Mesail-i Mühimme-i Hayatiye ve Sıhhiyeden Kısır Kadınlar* (Important Problems about Life and Health: Infertile Women) (Istanbul: Kader Matbaası, 1336 (1920)).

Avanzade Mehmed Süleyman (trans.), *Kız mı Oğlan mı?* (Is it a Girl or a Boy?) (Istanbul: Araks Matbaası, 1330 (1914)).

Aziz, 'Iskat-ı Cenin' (Abortion), *Mecmua-i Fünun*, 41 (December 1866), pp. 289–92.

Basiretçi Ali Efendi, 'Kadın Ebeler (Kabileler)' (Midwives), in *İstanbul Mektupları*, ed. N. Sağlam (Istanbul: Kitabevi, 2001), pp. 679–80.

Basiretçi, A., 'Şehir Mektubu, no. 157' (The City Letters, no: 157), *Basiret*, 2318 (13. Ra.1295/17 January 1878), pp. 2–3.

Debay, A., *Sıhhatnüma-yı İzdivac: Evleneceklerle Müteehhil ve Mücerred Bulunanlara Nasihat* (The Ways for Healthy Marriage: Advice for the Married, the Single and those Who Would Marry) , trans. Besim Ömer (Istanbul: Alem Matbaası, 1306, (1888/9)).

—, *Hygiène et physiologie du mariage; histoire naturelle et médicale de l'homme et de la femme mariés; dans ses plus curieux détails. Théorie nouvelle de la procréation mâle et femalle, stérilité, impuissance, imperfections génitales, moyens de les combattre. Hygiène spéciale de la femme enceinte et du nouveau-né* (Paris, E. Dentu, 1859).

Gebe Kalmamak İçin Ne Yapmalı? (The Precautions to Avoid Pregnancy) (Istanbul: Sevimli Ay Matbaası, 1927).

Halid Ziya (Uşaklıgil), *Haml-ü Vaz'ı Haml* (Pregnancy and Childbirth) (Istanbul: Mihran Matbaası, 1306, (1888/9)).

—, *Kanun ve Fenn-i Vilade* (The Laws and Science of Childbirth) ((Istanbul: Nişan Berberyan Matbaası, 1311 (1893)).

Halil Hamid, *Yeni Aile Rehberi* (The New Family Guide) (Istanbul : Hukuk Matbaası, 1919).

Hanım Kızlara (For the Young Girls) (Istanbul: A. Maviyan Şirket-i Mürettibiye Matbaası, 1304 (1887)).

Hasan Bedreddin Paşa, *Iskat-ı Cenin: Facia* (Abortion: A Tragedy) (Istanbul: 1290 (1873)).

Her Genç Kız Neler Bilmelidir? (What Should Every Young Girl Know?) (Istanbul: Sevimli Ay Matbaası, 1926).

Hüseyin Remzi, *Miratül-beyt. Hanımlara Yadigar* (A Heirloom for Women) (Istanbul, 1891).

—, *Sağdıç Rehber-i İzdivac* (Bestman Marriage Guide) (Istanbul: Artin Asaduryan Şirket-i Mürettibiye Matbaası, 1315 (1899)).

—, *Yadigâr-ı Remzi: Aile Hıfzı's-sıhhası* (Heirloom from Remzi: The Health of Family) (Istanbul: A. Asaduryan Şirket-i Mürettibiye Matbaası, 1900).

Kabile Rasiha, 'Yirmi Senelik Ebelik Hayatımda Neler Gördüm?' (What did I See in my Twenty Years of Midwifery Experience?), *Resimli Ay*, 29:21 (October 1925), pp. 43–6.

M. Faik, *Saadet-i Aile* (The Happiness of Family) (Istanbul: A. Asaduryan Şirket-i Mürettibiye Matbaası, 1316 (1899)).

Mehmed Süleyman Avanzade, *Gençlerde İstimna Bi-l-yed* (Masturbation among Young People) (Istanbul: Kader Matbaası, 1329, 1913).

—, *Yalnız Erkeklere Mahsus Adem-i İktidar* (Impotence Just for Men) (Istanbul: Kasbar Matbaası, 1330 (1914)).

—, *Yeni, Mükemmel, Son Rehber-i İzdivac* (New, Perfect, Latest Marriage Guide) (Istanbul: el-Adl Matbaası, 1338 (1922)).

Mustafa Safi, *Evlendirecek, Evlenecek ve Evlenmişlere Mahsus Saadet-i İzdivac* (The Happiness in Marriage for Those Who Would Marry Others, Who Would Get Married, and the Married) (Istanbul: Asır Matbaası, 1325 (1907/8)).

—, *Saadet-i İzdivac* (The Happiness in Marriage) (Istanbul: Asır Matbaası, 1325 (1907/8)).

Namık Kemal, 'Nüfus' (Population), *İbret*, 9 (19.R.1289/26 June 1872).

—, 'Iskat-ı Cenin' (Abortion), *Hadika*, 15 (27.N.1289/28 November 1872).

Necmeddin Sami, *Sevda Çiçekleri yahud İzdivacın Ehemmiyeti* (The Flowers of Love or the Importance of Marriage) (Istanbul: Kasbar Matbaası, 1312 (1895)).

Pierre Budin, *Seririyyat-ı Viladiyye dersleri* (The Lessons on Clinial Instruction of Child Birth), trans. Besim Ömer (Istanbul: Mekteb-i Tıbbiyye-i Şahane Matbaası, 1313 (1895/6)).

Redhouse, J. W., *Turkish and English Lexicon* (London: Oriental Literature Society, 1309 (1892)).

Salih Saim, *Ana Baba Nasihatları* (Advice for Parents) (Istanbul : Kasbar Matbaası, 1889).

Sedad Tosunpaşazade, *Muamelat-ı Zevciyede Adem-i İktidar* (Impotence in the Relationship of the Couples) (Istanbul: Şems Matbaası, 1328 (1912)).

Şemseddin Sami, *Kamus-ı Türki,* (Turkish Dictionary) (Dersaadet: İkdam Matbaası, 1317 (1899)).

Seyyid Tahir, *Vaz'ı Haml: İbtia-ı Hamil, Kabilenin Vazifesi, Cenin* (Childbirth: The Beginning of Pregnancy, the Duties of the Midwife, Embryo and Foetus) (Istanbul: Şems Matbaası, 1331 (1915)).

Skanzoni, *Fenn-i Vilade* (The Science of Birth) (Istanbul: Mekteb-i Tıbbiye-i Şahane Matbaası, 1298 (1880/1)).

Books, Articles and Dissertations

Abdülaziz Bey, *Osmanlı Adet, Merasim ve Tabirleri/Adat ve Merasim-i Kadime, Tabirat ve Muamelat-i Kavmiye-i Osmaniye* (Ottoman Customs, Ceremonies and Idioms), ed. K. Arısan and D. A. Günay (Istanbul: Tarih Vakfı Yurt Yayınları, 1995).

Abou-El-Haj, R. A., *Formation of the Modern State: The Ottoman Empire, Sixteenth to Eighteenth Centuries* (Syracuse, NY: Syracuse University Press, 2005).

Abugideiri, H., 'Egyptian Women and the Science Question: Gender in the Making of Colonized Medicine, 1893–1929' (PhD dissertation, Georgetown University, 2001).

—, 'The Scientisation of Culture: Colonial Medicine's Construction of Egyptian Womanhood, 1893–1929', *Gender & History*, 16:1 (2004), pp. 83–9.

Agmon, I., 'Women, Class, and Gender: Muslim Jaffa and Haifa at the Turn of the 20th Century', *International Journal of Middle East Studies*, 30:4 (1998), pp. 477–500.

—, *Family & Court: Legal Culture and Modernity in Late Ottoman Palestine* (Syracuse, NY: Syracuse University Press, 2006).

Ahmad, F., *The Young Turks; The Committee of Union and Progress in Turkish Politics* (Oxford: Clarendon Press, 1969).

Ak, B., and A. Ataç (eds), *Osmanlı Devleti'nde Sağlık Hizmetleri Sempozyumu* (The Health Services in the Ottoman State Symposium) (Ankara: Sağlık Bakanlığı, 2000).

Akgündüz, A., *Mukayeseli İslam ve Osmanlı Hukuku Külliyatı* (Comparative Complete Works on Islamic and Ottoman Law) (Diyarbakır: Dicle Üniversitesi Hukuk Fakültesi Yayınları, 1986).

—, *Şer'iye Sicilleri: Mahiyeti, Toplu Kataloğu ve Seçme Hükümler* (Court Records: Contents, Complete Catalogue and Selective Verdicts) (Istanbul: Türk Dünyası Araştırmaları Vakfı, 1988).

Akkan, A., 'Dr. Besim Ömer Paşa (Akalın)' (Doctor Besim Ömer Paşa (Akalın)), *Mimar Sinan*, 6 (1992), pp. 15–20.

Akşit, E. E., 'Girls' Education and the Paradoxes of Modernity and Nationalism in the Late Ottoman Empire and the Early Turkish Republic' (PhD Dissertation, Binghamton University, 2004).

—, 'Geç Osmanlı ve Cumhuriyet Dönemlerinde Nüfus Kontrolü Yaklaşımları' (The Approaches to Population Control in the Late Ottoman and Early Republican Periods), *Toplum ve Bilim*, 118 (2010), pp. 179–97.

Aktaş, N. et al., *Başbakanlık Osmanlı Arşivi Rehberi* (The Guide for Prime Ministry Ottoman Archive) (Istanbul: Başbakanlık Devlet Arşivleri Genel Müdürlüğü Osmanlı Arşivi Daire Başkanlığı, 2000).

Akyıldız, A., *Tanzimat Dönemi Osmanlı Merkez Teşkilatında Reform* (Reform of the Ottoman Central Administration during the Tanzimat Period) (Istanbul: Eren, 1993).

—, *Osmanlı Bürokrasisi ve Modernleşme* (Ottoman Bureaucracy and Modernization) (Istanbul: İletişim Yayınevi, 2004).

Altıntaş, A., 'Türkiye'de Ebelik Eğitimi' (Midwifery Education in Turkey), in H. Hatemi and A. Altıntaş (eds), *Türk Tıp Eğitiminin Önemli Adımları* (Important Steps of Turkish Medical Education) (Istanbul: CSA Global Publishing, 2006), pp. 156–60.

Altınöz, V. D., 'The Ottoman Women's Movement: Women's Press, Magazines, Journals, and Newspapers from 1875 to 1923' (MA thesis, University of Miami, 2003).

Anderson, B., *Imagined Communities: Reflections on the Origin and Spread of Nationalism* (London: Verso, 1991).

Aprahamian, S., and V. Rowe (eds), *Ottoman Women's Movements and Print Cultures* (Austin, TX: University of Texas Press, forthcoming).

Arısan, K., *Doğum Yardımının Dünü, Bugünü ve Bizde Ev-Saray Doğumlarıyla İlgili Gelenekler* (The Present and Past of Assistance during Childbirth, The Customs about Childbirth in Houses-Palaces) (Istanbul: Istanbul Üniversitesi Tıp Fakültesi, 1980).

—, 'Geçen Yüzyılda İstanbul'da Ebeler ve Doğum', in *Türk Tıp Tarihi Kongresi, İstanbul (17–19 Şubat 1988)* (The Proceeding of 1st Turkish History of Medicine Congress (17–19 February 1988) (Ankara: Türk Tarih Kurumu, 1992), pp. 253–259.

Aydın, C., 'Mecmua-i Fünun ve Mecmua-i Ulum Dergilerinin Medeniyet ve Bilim Anlayışı' (The Notions of Civilization and Science of the Journals Mecmua-i Fünun and Mecmua-i Ulum) (MA Thesis, Istanbul University, 1995).

Aydın, M., 'Sultan II. Mahmud Döneminde Yapılan Nüfus Tahrirleri' (The Population Censuses during the Period of Sultan Mahmud II), in *Sultan II. Mahmud ve Reformları Semineri: 28–30 Haziran 1989* (The Seminars on Sultan Mahmud II and his Reforms: 28–30 June 1989) (Istanbul: İstanbul Üniversitesi Edebiyat Fakültesi Tarih Araştırmaları Enstitüsü, 1990), pp. 81–106.

Aykut Türker, E., 'Alternative Claims on Justice and Law: Rural Arson and Poison Murder in the 19th Century Ottoman Empire' (PhD dissertation, Boğaziçi University, 2011).

Aynur, H., 'Malumatçı Baba Tahir' ('Baba Tahir, [Publisher] of Malumat), *Toplumsal Tarih*, 128 (2004), pp. 62–5.

Baer, M., 'Islamic Conversion Narratives of Women: Social Change and Gendered Religious Hierarchy in Early Modern Ottoman İstanbul', *Gender & History*, 16:2 (2004), pp. 425–58.

—, 'Manliness, Male Virtue and History Writing at the Seventeenth-Century Ottoman Court', *Gender & History*, 20:1 (2008), pp. 128–48.

Baldry, J., 'The Ottoman Quarantine Station on Karaman Island, 1881–1914', *Studies in History of Medicine*, 2 (1978), pp. 3–138.

Balıkhane Nazırı Ali Rıza Bey, *Bir Zamanlar İstanbul* (Istanbul Once Upon a Time) (Tercüman 1001 Temel Eser, undated).

Balsoy, G., 'Advices to Pregnant Women: Changing Conceptions of Pregnancy and Birth in the Ottoman Empire in the Late Nineteenth Century', in ed. T. D. Sechel, *Medicine Within and Between the Habsburg and Ottoman Empires, 18th–19th centuries* (Bochum: Verlag, 2010), pp. 149–64.

Banks, A. C., *Birth Chairs, Midwives and Medicine* (Jackson, MS: University Press of Mississippi, 1999).

Basiretçi Ali Efendi., 'Kadın Ebeler (Kabileler)' (Midwives), in N. Sağlam, *İstanbul Mektupları* (Istanbul: Kitabevi, 2001), pp. 679–80.

Belger, N. R., 'Türk Kadınının ve Çocuğunun Minnettar Olduğu Büyük Adam' (The Great Man that Turkish Women and Children are Grateful to), *Akşam* (19 March 1945).

Berktay, H., *Cumhuriyet İdeolojisi ve Fuat Köprülü* (The Ideology of the Republic and Fuat Köprülü) (Istanbul: Kaynak Yayınları, 1983).

Bowen, D. L., 'Abortion, Islam, and the 1994 Cairo Population Conference', *International Journal of Middle East Studies*, 29:2 (1997), pp. 161–84.

Bozkurt, A., '93 Harbi Eşiğinde Selanik'te Bir Kadın Dergisi: Ayine (1875–1876)' (A Women's Journal in Thessaloniki before the War of '93: Ayine (1875-1876)), *Kebikeç*, 19 (2005), pp. 73–97.

Brockopp, J. E., *Islamic Ethics of Life: Abortion, War, and Euthanasia* (Columbia, SC: University of South Carolina Press, 2003).

Broomhall, S., ''Women's Little Secrets': Defining the Boundaries of Reproductive Knowledge in Sixteenth Century', *Social History of Medicine*, 15:1 (2002), pp. 1–15.

Buturovic, A., and I. C. Schick (eds), *Women in the Ottoman Balkans: Gender, Culture and History* (London: I. B. Tauris, 2007).

Çadırcı, M., 'Tanzimat Döneminde Çıkarılan Men'i Mürur ve Pasaport Nizamnameleri' (The Regulations of Passport and Transit Bans during the Tanzimat Period), *Belgeler*, 15:19 (1993), pp. 169–81.

Çakır, C., *Tanzimat Dönemi Osmanlı Maliyesi* (Ottoman Finace during the Tanzimat Period) (Istanbul: Küre Yayınları, 2001).

Çakır, S., *Osmanlı Kadın Hareketi* (Ottoman Women's Movement) (Istanbul: Metis Yayınları, 1994).

Camiscioli, E., 'Producing Citizens, Reproducing the "French Race": Immigration, Demography, and Pronatalism in Early Twentieth-Century France', *Gender & History*, 13:3 (Fall 2001), pp. 593–621.

Cemiloğlu, M., *Halk Hikayelerinde Doğum Motifi* (Patterns of Childbirth in Folk Tales) (Bursa: Uludağ Üniversitesi Güçlendirme Vakfı, 1999).

Çetinsaya, G., 'Abdülhamit'i Anlamak: 19. Yüzyıl Tarihçiliğine Bir Bakış'(Understanding Abdülhamit: An Overview of the Historiography of 19th Century), in *Sosyal Bilimleri Yeniden Düşünmek: Toplum Bilim ve Defter Dergileri Sempozyum Bildirgeleri* (Rethinking the Social Sciences: The Proceedings of Toplum ve Bilim and Defter Journals' Symposium) (Istanbul: Metis, 1998), pp. 137–46.

Cole, J. H., *The Power of Large Numbers: Population, Politics, and Gender in Nineteenth-Century France* (Ithaca, NY: Cornell University Press, 2000).

Cuno, K. M., and M. J. Reimer, 'The Census Registers of Nineteenth-Century Egypt: A New Source for Social Historians', *British Journal of Middle Eastern Studies*, 24:2 (1997), pp. 193–216.

Davin, A., 'Imperialism and Motherhood', in F. Cooper and A. L. Stoler (eds), *Tensions of Empire: Colonial Cultures in a Bourgeois World* (Berkeley, CA: University of California Press, 1997), pp. 87–151.

Davis, F., *The Ottoman Lady: A Social History From 1718 to 1918* (Westport, CT: Greenwood Press, 1986).

Delaney, C., *The Seed and the Soil: Gender and Cosmology in Turkish Village* (Berkeley, CA: University of California, 1991).

Delice, S., 'Friendship, Sociability, and Masculinity in the Ottoman Empire: An Essay Confronting the Ghosts of Historicism', *New Perspectives on Turkey*, 42 (Spring 2010), pp. 103–25.

Demirci, T., 'Body, Disease and Late Ottoman Literature: Debates on Ottoman Muslim Family in the Tanzimat Period (1839–1908)' (PhD Dissertation, Bilkent University, 2008).

Demirci, T., and S. A. Somel, 'Women's Bodies, Demography, and Public Health: Abortion Policy and Perspectives in the Ottoman Empire of the Nineteenth Century', *Journal of the History of Sexuality*, 17:3 (2008), pp. 377–420.

Demirdirek, A., *Osmanlı Kadınlarının Hayat Hakkı Arayışının Bir Hikayesi* (A Story of Ottoman Women's Search for their Rights for Living) (Ankara: İmge Kitabevi, 1993).

Deringil, S., 'New Approaches to the Study of the Ottoman Nineteenth Century', in Ç. Kafesçioğlu and L. Thys-Şenocak (eds), *Aptullah Kuran için Yazılar* (Istanbul: YKY, 1999).

—, *The Well-Protected Domains: Ideology and the Legitimation of Power in the Ottoman Empire, 1876–1909* (London: I. B. Tauris, 1999).

Dinç, F. G., 'Ignorant, Dirty, Superstitious Crones: Degrading of Midwifery and Midwives in Modern Turkey' (MA Thesis, Istanbul Bilgi University, 2011).

Dirican, R., 'Türkiye'de Ebeliğin Kısa Tarihçesi' (A Short History of Midwifery in Turkey), *Dirim*, 1–2 (1973).

Doumani, B. (ed.), 'The Political Economy of Population Counts in Ottoman Palestine: Nablus, circa 1850', *International Journal of Middle East Studies*, 26:1 (1994), pp. 1–17.

—, *Family History in the Middle East: Household, Property, and Gender*. (Albany, NY: University of New York Press, 2003).

Duben, A., and C. Behar, *İstanbul Households: Marriage, Family and Fertility, 1880–1940* (New York: Cambridge University Press, 2002).

Duden, B., *The Woman Beneath the Skin: A Doctor's Patients in Eighteenth-century*, trans. T. Dunlap. (Cambridge, MA: Harvard University Press, 1991).

—, *Disembodying Women: Perspectives on Pregnancy and the Unborn*, trans. L. Hoinacki (Cambridge, MA: Harvard University Press, 1993).

Dündar, F., *Modern Türkiye'nin Şifresi: İttihat ve Terakki'nin Etnisite Mühendisliği (1913–1918)* (The Crypto of Modern Turkey: The Ethnicity Engineering of [the Committee of] Union and Progress) (Istanbul: İletişim Yayınevi, 2008).

Dursun, S., 'Population Policies of the Ottoman State in the Tanzimat Era: 1840–1870' (MA Thesis, Sabancı University, 2001).

Dye, N. S., 'History of Childbirth in America', *Signs, Women: Sex and Sexuality, Part 2*, 6:1 (1980), pp. 97–108.

Ehrenreich, B., and D. English, *Witches, Midwives and Nurses: A History of Women Healers* (New York, 1973).

Elmacı, N., 'Doğum Gelenekleri: Bakacak Köyünün Dünü ve Bugünü'(The Customs of Childbirth: The Past and Present of Village Bakacak), *Folklor Edebiyat*, 30:2 (2002).

Engelstein, L., *The Keys to Happiness: Sex and the Search for Modernity in Fin-de-Siècle Russia* (Ithaca, NY: Cornell University Press, 1992).

Erden, F., *Türk Hekimleri Biyografisi* (The Bibliography of Turkish Doctors) (Istanbul: Cituri Biraderler Basımevi, 1948).

Ergin, O. N., *Mecelle-i Umur-u Belediyye* (Civil Code of Municipal Works), 6 volumes (Istanbul: İstanbul Büyükşehir Belediyesi Kültür İşleri Daire Başkanlığı, 1995), vol. 6.

Ersanlı, B., *İktidar ve Tarih: Türkiye'de "Resmi Tarih" Tezinin Oluşumu (1929–1937)* (Power and History: The Formation of 'Official History' in Turkey) (Istanbul: İletişim Yayınevi, 2003).

Evenden, D., *The Midwives of Seventeenth Century London* (Cambridge: Cambridge University Press, 2000).

Eyüboğlu, İ. Z., *Anadolu İnançları Anadolu Mitologisi: İnanç-Söylence Bağlantısı* (Anatolian Beliefs Anatolian Mythology: The Links between Beliefs and Tales) (Istanbul: Geçit Kitabevi, 1987).

Fahmy, K., *All the Pasha's Men: Mehmed Ali, his Army, and the Making of Modern Egypt* (Cambridge: Cambridge University Press, 1997).

—, 'Women, Medicine and Power in Nineteenth-Century Egypt', in L. Abou-Lughod (ed.), *Remaking Women: Feminism and Modernity in the Middle East* (Princeton, NJ: Princeton University Press, 1998).

Findley, C. V., *Bureaucratic Reform in the Ottoman Empire: The Sublime Porte, 1789–1922* (Princeton, NJ: Princeton University Press, 1980).

Fortna, B., *Imperial Classroom: Islam the State and Education in the Late Ottoman Empire* (New York: Oxford University Press, 2003).

Frierson, E., 'Unimagined Communities: Women and Education in the Late-Ottoman Empire, 1876–1909', *Critical Matrix, The Princeton Journal of Women, Gender, and Culture*, 9:2 (1995), pp. 55–90.

—, 'Women in Ottoman Intellectual History', in E. Özdalga (ed.), *Late Ottoman Society: The Intellectual Heritage* (New York: Routledge-Curzon, 2005), pp. 135–62.

Genç, M., and E. Özvar (eds), *Osmanlı Maliyesi Kurumlar ve Bütçeler* (Ottoman Finance Institutions and Budgets) (Istanbul: Osmanlı Bankası Arşiv ve Araştırma Merkezi, 2006).

Greil, A. L., 'Infertile Bodies: Medicalization, Metaphor, and Agency', in M. Inhorn and F. Van Balen (eds), *Infertility Around the Globe* (Berkeley, CA: University of California Press, 2002), pp. 101–19.

Green, M. H., 'From "Diseases of Women" to "Secrets of Women": The Transformation of Gynecological Literature in the Later Middle Ages'. *Journal of Medieval and Early Modern Studies*, 30:1 (2000), pp. 5–39.

—, 'Gendering the History of Women's Healthcare', *Gender & History* 20:3 (2008), pp. 487–518.

Grossman, A., *Reforming Sex: The German Movement for Birth Control and Abortion Reform 1920–1950* (New York: Oxford University Press, 1995).

Gülsoy, U., *Osmanlı Gayrimüslimlerinin Askerlik Serüveni* (The History of Military Service of the Ottoman non-Muslims) (Istanbul: Simurg Yayınevi, 2000).

Gündüz, F. S., 'Osmanlı Devleti'nin Son Dönemlerinde Kadınlara Mahsus bir Hastane: Haseki (A Hospital for Women in the Final Periods of Ottoman State: Haseki), *Yeni Tıp Tarihi Araştırmaları* (New Researches on History of Medicine), 5 (1999), pp. 95–112.

Gürsoy, A., 'Abortion in Turkey: A Matter of State, Family or Individual Decision', *Social Science and Medicine*, 42:4 (1996), pp. 531–42.

Güvenç Salgırlı, S., 'Eugenics as Science of the Social: A Case from 1930s Istanbul' (PhD Dissertation, Binghamton University, 2009).

Hanioğlu, Ş., 'Osmanlıcılık' (Ottomanism), in *Tanzimattan Cumhuriyete Türkiye Ansiklopedisi* (Encyclopaedia of Turkey from Tanzimat to the Republic) , 6 vols (Istanbul: İletişim Yayınevi, 1985), vol. 5, pp. 1389–93.

—, *The Young Turks in Opposition* (New York: Oxford University Press, 1995).

—, *Preparation for a Revolution: The Young Turks, 1902–1908* (New York: Oxford University Press, 2001).

Harley, D., 'Historians as Demonologists: The Myth of the Midwife-Witch', *Social History of Medicine*, 3 (1990), pp. 1–26.

–, 'Provincial Midwives in England: 1660–1760', in H. Marland (ed.), *The Art of Midwifery: Early Modern Midwives in Europe* (London: Routledge, 1994).

Hatem, M. F., 'The Professionalization of Health and the Control of Women's Bodies as Modern Governmentalities in Nineteenth-Century Egypt', in M. C. Zilfi (ed.), *Women in the Ottoman Empire: Middle Eastern Women in the Early Modern Era* (Brill, 1997), pp. 66–80.

Helimoğlu, M. Y., *Diyarbakır Efsaneleri; Derleme-Araştırma-İnceleme* (The Myths of Diyarbakır: Collections-Survey-Examination) (Ankara: Doruk, 1993).

Homei, A., 'Sanba and their Clients: Midwives and the Medicalization of Childbirth in Japan', in B. Mortimer and S. McGann (eds), *New Directions in the History of Nursing* (London: Routledge, 2005), pp. 68–85.

—, 'Birth Attendants in Meiji Japan: The Rise of a Medical Birth Model and the New Division of Labour', *Social History of Medicine*, 19:3 (2006), pp. 407–24.

Hot, İ., 'Besim Ömer Paşanın Anne ve Çocuk Sağlığı Açısından Ülkemiz Nüfus Meselesi Hakkındaki Görüşleri' (The Ideas of Besim Ömer Paşa on the Population of our Country from the Perspective of the Health of Mothers and Children) (MA Thesis, Istanbul University, 1996).

—, 'Besim Ömer Akalın (1862–1940)', *Yeni Tıp Tarihi Araştırmaları* (New Researches on History of Medicine), 2–3 (1996–7), pp. 213–32.

Imber, C., *Ebu's-Su'ud: The Islamic Legal Tradition* (Stanford, CA: Stanford University Press, 1997).

Ilyasoğlu, A., and D. İnsel, 'Kadın Dergilerinin Evrimi' (The Evolution of Women's Journals), in *Türkiye'de Dergiler, Ansiklopediler (1849–1984)* (Journals and Encyclopaedias in Turkey) (Istanbul: Gelişim Yayınları, 1984).

Inal, İbnü'l Emin Mahmut Kemal, *Son Asır Türk Şairleri* (The Turkish Poets of the Last Century) (Istanbul: Türk Tarih Encümeni Külliyatı, 1930).

Inalcık, H., 'Application of the Tanzimat and its Social Effects', *Archivum Ottomanicum*, 5 (1973), pp. 97–128.

Inalcık, H., and M. Seyitdanlıoğlu (eds), *Tanzimat: Değişim Sürecinde Osmanlı İmparatorluğu* (Tanzimat: Ottoman Empire in the Process of Change) (Istanbul: Phoenix, 2006).

Işıl, Y, 'Bir Aydınlanma Hareketi Olarak Mecmua-iFünun' (Mecmua-i Fünun as a Movement of Enlightenment) (MA Thesis, Istanbul University, 1986).

Janet B., 'Care or Cure? Childbirth Practices in Nineteenth Century America', *Feminist Studies*, 4:2 (1978), pp. 92–9.

Kahya, E., and A. D. Erdemir, *Medicine in the Ottoman Empire (and Other Scientific Developments)* (Istanbul: Nobel Tıp Kitabevleri, 1997).

—, *Bilimin Işığında Osmanlıdan Cumhuriyete Tıp ve Sağlık Kurumları* (The Institutions of Medicine and Health from the Ottomans to the Republic in the Light of Science) (Ankara: Türkiye Diyanet Vakfı Yayınları, 2000).

—, *Science of Medicine in the Ottoman Empire* (Pakistan: Hamdar Foundation, 2003).

—, *Medical Studies and Institutions in the Ottoman Empire: With Brief Information about the Scientific Studies* (Ankara: Nobel Yayın Dağıtım Tic. Ltd. Şti., 2008).

Karakaya-Stump, A., 'Debating Progress in a 'Serious Newspaper for Muslim Women': The Periodical Kadın of the Post-revolutionary Salonica, 1908–1909', *British Journal of Middle Eastern Studies*, 30:2 (2003), pp. 155–81.

Karal, E. Z., *Osmanlı İmparatorluğu'nda İlk Nüfus Sayımı 1831* (The First Population Census in the Ottoman Empire 1831) (Ankara: Başvekalet İstatistik Umum Müdürlüğü, 1943).

—, *Osmanlı Tarihi, 1. Cilt Nizam-ı Cedid ve Tanzimat Devirleri (1789–1856)* (The History of the Ottomans: The Period of Nizam-i Cedid and Tanzimat) (Ankara: Türk Tarih Kurumu, 1988).

Karpat, K., 'The Transformation of the Ottoman State, 1789–1908', *International Journal of Middle East Studies*, 3:3 (1972), pp. 243–81.

—, 'Ottoman Population Records and the Census of 1881/82–1893', *International Journal of Middle East Studies*, 9:3 (1978), pp. 237–74.

—, *Ottoman Population, 1830–1914* (Madison, WI: University of Wisconsin Press, 1985).

Kaya, A. Y., 'Vergilendirmenin Ekonomi Politiği: 19. Yüzyıl Ortasında İzmir Kadastrosu' (The Political Economy of Taxation: Land Survey of Izmir in mid-19th Century) , *İzmir'in Dünden Bugüne Sosyal ve Ekonomik Gelişimi Konferansı Bildirileri* (The Proceedings of The Conference of the Social and Economic Development of Izmir from Yesterday to Today) (İzmir: İzmir Ekonomi Üniversitesi, İzmir İktisat Kongresi Araştırma Merkezi, 2007).

—, '19. Yüzyıl Ortasında İzmir'de Mülkiyet, Emniyet ve Zabtiyeler'(Private Property, Security and the Police in Izmir in mid-Nineteenth Century), in N. Lévy, N. Özbek and A. Toumarkine (eds), *Jandarma ve Polis: Fransız ve Osmanlı Tarihçiliği Çapraz Bakışlar* (Gendarmary and the Police: Comparative Approaches to French and Ottoman Historiographies) (Istanbul: Tarih Vakfı, 2009).

Kazancıgil, A., 'Ölümünün 40. Yılında Besim Ömer Paşa (1863–1940)' (Besim Ömer Paşa on his 40th Anniversary), *Dirim* (Life), 55 (1980), pp. 9–10.

Keddie, N., and B. Baron (eds), *Women in Middle Eastern History: Shifting Boundaries in Sex and Gender* (New Haven, CT: Yale University Press, 1991).

Keskin, R. M., and S. Sağlık, 'Türkiyede Viladiye ve Nisaiye Tarihinden bir Hulasa' (Brief Ideas on the History of Obstetrics and Gynaecology in Turkey), *Türk Tıp Tarihi Arkivi* (Turkish History of Medicine Archive) (1939), pp. 101–6.

Kılıç Denman, F., 'İkinci Meşrutiyet Döneminde bir Jön Türk Dergisi: "Kadın"' (A Young Turk Magazine in the Second Constitutional Period: Kadın) (Istanbul: Libra Yayıncılık, 2010).

Kılıç, F., 'Kadın: A Young Turk Magazine in the Second Constitutional Period (1908–1909)' (MA thesis, Boğaziçi University, 2005).

Kılınç, H., 'Isolating the Subject: Cholera, Control and Sanitary Discourse in the İstanbul International Sanitary Conference of 1866' (MA Thesis, Boğaziçi University, 2005).

Kırlı, C., 'Kahvehaneler ve Hafiyeler: 19. Yüzyıl Ortalarında Osmanlı'da Sosyal Kontrol'(Coffeehouses and Spies: Social Control in Ottoman Society during mid-19th Century), *Toplum ve Bilim* (Society and Science), 83 (2000), pp. 58–79.

—, 'The Struggle Over Space: Coffeehouses of Ottoman İstanbul 1780–1845' (PhD dissertation, Binghamton University, 2000).

—, 'A Profile of the Labor Force in Early Nineteenth-Century Istanbul', *International Labor and Working Class History*, 60 (2001), pp. 125–40.

—, 'Coffeehouses: Public Opinion in the Nineteenth Century Ottoman Empire', in A. Salvatore and D. F. Eickelman (eds), *Public Islam and the Common Good* (Boston, MA: Brill, 2004).

—, 'Yolsuzluğun İcadı: 1840 Ceza Kanunu, İktidar ve Bürokrasi' (The Invention of Corruption: The 1840 Criminal Law, Power and Bureaucracy), *Tarih ve Toplum Yeni Yaklaşımlar* (History and Society New Approaches), 4 (2006), pp. 45–119.

Köker, A. H. (ed.), *Doğum ve Ebelik Tarihi Kongresi, 14 Mart, 1997* (The History of Childbirth and Midwifery Congress) (Kayseri: Kayseri Erciyes Üniversitesi Gevher Nesibi Tıp Tarihi Enstitüsü, 1997).

Kozma, L., 'Women on the Margins and Legal Reform in Late Nineteenth Century Egypt, 1850–1882' (PhD dissertation, New York University, 2006).

Kukla, R., *Mass Hysteria: Medicine, Culture, and Mothers' Bodies* (Lanham, MD: Rowman and Littlefield, 2005).

Kurnaz, Ş., *Cumhuriyet Öncesinde Türk Kadını: 1839–1923* (Turkish Woman Before the Republic: 1839–1923) (Ankara: Başbakanlık Aile Araştırma Kurumu, 1991).

Leavitt, J. W., '"Science" Enters the Birthing Room: Obstetrics in America since the Eighteenth Century', *Journal of American History*, 70:2 (1983), pp. 281–304.

—, *Brought to Bed: Child Bearing in America, 1750–1950* (New York: Oxford University Press, 1986).

Lindemann, M., 'Professionals? Sisters? Rivals? Midwives in Braunschweig, 1750–1800', in H. Marland (ed.), *The Art of Midwifery: Early Modern Midwives in Europe* (London: Routledge, 1994).

—, *Medicine and Society in Early Modern Europe* (Cambridge: Cambridge University Press, 1999).

Loudin, I., 'Deaths in Childbed from the Eighteenth Century to 1935', *Medical History* 30 (1986), pp. 1–41.

—, *Death in Childbirth: An International Study of Maternal Care and Maternal Mortality, 1800–1950* (Oxford: Oxford University Press, 1992).

Maksudyan, N., 'Hearing the Voiceless-Seeing the Invisible: Orphans and Destitute Children as Actors of Social, Economic, and Political History in the Late Ottoman Empire' (PhD dissertation, Sabancı University, 2008).

—, '"This Time Women as Well Got Involved in Politics!": Nineteenth Century Ottoman Women's Organizations and Political Agency', in S. Aprahamian and V. Rowe (eds), *Ottoman Women's Movements and Print Cultures* (Austin, TX: University of Texas Press, forthcoming).

Mardin, Ş., *The Genesis of Young Ottoman Thought: A Study in the Modernization of Turkish Political Ideas* (Syracuse, NY: Syracuse University Press, 2000).

Marland, H. (ed.), *The Art of Midwifery: Early Modern Midwives in Europe* (London: Routledge, 1994).

Matossian, M. K., and S. Hoogasian Villa, *1914 Öncesi Ermeni Köy Hayatı* (Armenian Village Life before 1914), trans. A. Yılmaz (Istanbul: Aras Yayıncılık, 2006).

McIntosh, T., 'Profession, Skill, or Domestic Duty? Midwifery in Sheffield, 1881–1936'. *Social History of Medicine*, 11:3 (1998), pp. 403–20.

McLaren, A., 'Abortion in England, 1890–1914', *Victorian Studies* 20:4 (1977), pp. 379–401.

—, 'Abortion in France: Women and the Regulation of Family Size, 1800-1914', *French Historical Studies*, 10:3 (1978), pp. 461–85.

—, *Reproductive Rituals: The Perception of Fertility in England from the Sixteenth to the Nineteenth Century* (London: Methuen, 1984).

Miller, R., 'Politicizing Reproduction in Comparative Perspective: Ottoman, Turkish, and French Approaches to Abortion Law', *Hawwa*, 5:1 (2007), pp. 73–89.

—, 'Rights, Reproduction, Sexuality, and Citizenship in the Ottoman Empire and Turkey', *Signs*, 32:2 (2007), pp. 347–75.

—, *The Limits of Bodily Integrity: Abortion, Adultery, and Rape Legislation in Comparative Perspective* (Aldershot: Ashgate, 2007).

Montagu, L. M. W., *The Complete Letters of Lady Mary Wortley Montegu: 1708–1720* (Oxford: Oxford University Press, 1967).

Moscucci, O., *The Science of Woman: Gynaecology and Gender in England, 1800–1929.* (Cambridge: Cambridge University Press, 1990).

Mossensohn, M. S., 'Health as a Social Agent in Ottoman Patronage and Authority', *New Perspectives on Turkey*, 37 (2007), pp. 147–75.

—, 'Tale of Two Discourses: The Historiography of Ottoman-Muslim Medicine', *Social History of Medicine*, 21:1(2008), pp. 1–12.

Oktar, T., *Osmanlı Toplumunda Kadının Çalışma Yaşamı, Osmanlı Kadınları Çalıştırma Cemiyet-i İslamiyesi* (The Professional Life of Women in Ottoman Society, Ottoman Islamic Society for Employing the Women) (Istanbul: Bilim Teknik Yayınevi, 1998).

Olgun, K., 'Osmanlı Devletinde Nüfusu Arttırma Politikası Çerçevesinde Iskat-ı Ceninin (Kürtaj) Yasaklanması' (The Ban of Abortion as Part of the Attempt to Icrease Population of the Ottoman State), in N. Sarı (ed.), *Uluslararası Tıp Tarihi Kongresi* (International Congress of History of Medicine) (Ankara: Türk Tarih Kurumu, 2005).

Onur, A. A., 'Büyük Alim ve Tıp Kahramanı, Besim Ömer Akalın'(The Big Man of Science and Hero of Medicine, Besim Ömer Akalın), in *Türk Ginekoloji Arşivi* (Turkish Archive of Gynaecology), 24:25 (1940), pp. 1177–80.

Ortaylı, İ., *İmparatorluğun En Uzun Yüzyılı* (The Longest Century of the Empire) (Istanbul: Hil Yayınevi, 1983).

—, *Tanzimat Devrinde Osmanlı Mahalli İdareleri: 1840–1880* (The Local Administrations during Tanzimat period: 1840-1880) (Ankara: Türk Tarih Kurumu, 2000).

Ozbay, F., 'Türkiye'de Ulus-Devlet, Gözetim ve Nüfus Bilgisi' (National State, Surveilance and Population Information in Turkey), *Toplum ve Bilim* (Soceity and Science) 118 (2010), pp. 165–78.

Ozbek, M., 'The Regulation of Prostitution in Beyoglu (1875–1915)', *Middle Eastern Studies*, 46:4 (January 2010), pp. 555–68.

Ozbek, N., *Osmanlı İmparatorluğu'nda Sosyal Devlet, Siyaset, İktidar ve Meşruiyet, 1876–1914* (Social Welfare, Politics, Power and Legitimacy in the Ottoman Empire, 1876-1914) (Istanbul: İletişim Yayınevi, 2002).

—, 'Imperial Gifts and Sultanic Legitimation During the Reign of Sultan Abdülhamid II, 1876-1909', in M. Ener, A. Singer and M. Bonner (eds), *Poverty and Charity in the Middle Eastern Contexts* (Albany, NY: University of New York Press, 2003).

—, 'Modernite, Tarih ve İdeoloji: II. Abdülhamid Dönemi Tarihçiliği Üzerine Bir Değerlendirme', *Türkiye Araştırmaları Literatür Dergisi*, 2:1 (2004), pp. 71–90.

—, 'Philanthropic Activity, Ottoman Patriotism and the Hamidian Regime, 1876–1909', *International Journal of Middle East Studies*, 37:1 (2005), pp. 59–81.

—, 'Defining the Public Sphere during the Late Ottoman Empire: War, Mass Mobilization and the Young Turk Regime (1908–18)', *Middle Eastern Studies*, 43:5 (2007), pp. 795–809.

Ozden, A. M., *Doktor Besim Ömer Akalın* (Doctor Besim Ömer Akalın) (Istanbul: Ahmet İhsan Matbaası, 1941).

Oztürk, M., 'Osmanlı Döneminde Iskat-ı Cenin Yeri ve Hükmü' (The Statue and Importance of Abrotion in Late Ottoman Period), *Fırat Üniversitesi Dergisi (Sosyal Bilimler)* (Journal of Fırat University (Social Sciences)), 1:1 (1987), pp. 199–208.

Ozvar, E., *Osmanlı Maliyesinde Malikane Uygulaması* (Tax Farming Practice in Ottoman Finance) (Istanbul: Kitabevi, 2003).

Palairet, M., *The Balkan Economies, c. 1800–1914. Evolution Without Development* (Cambridge: Cambridge University Press, 1997).

Pamuk, Ş., *The Ottoman Empire and European Capitalism, 1820–1913* (Cambridge: Cambridge University Press, 1987).

—, *Osmanlı-Türkiye İktisadi Tarihi, 1500–1914* (Ottoman-Turkish History of Economics, 1500-1914) (Istanbul: İletişim Yayınevi, 2005).

Patriarca, S., *Numbers and Nationhood: Writing Statistics in Nineteenth-Century Italy* (Cambridge: Cambridge University Press, 1996).

Pedersen, J. E., 'Regulating Abortion and Birth Control: Gender, Medicine, and Republican Politics in France, 1870–1920', *French Historical Studies*, 19:3 (1996), pp. 673–98.

Peirce, L., *Morality Tales: Law and Gender in the Ottoman Court of Aintab* (Berkeley, CA: University of California Press, 2003).

Pollock, L. A., 'Embarking on a Rough Passage: The Experience of Maternity in Early Modern Society', in D. MacLaren and V. A. Fildes (eds), *Women as Mothers in Pre-industrial England: Essays in Memory of Dorothy McLaren* (London: Routledge, 1990), pp. 39–67.

Poovey, M., 'Scenes of an Indelicate Character: The Medical "Treatment" of Victorian Women', *Representations*, 14, *The Making of the Modern Body: Sexuality and Society in the Nineteenth Century* (1986), pp. 137–68.

Quataert, D., *Ottoman Manufacturing in the Age of Industrial Revolution* (Cambridge: Cambridge University Press, 1993).

—, 'The Age of Reforms, 1812–1914', in H. İnalcık and D. Quataert (eds), *An Economic and Social History of the Ottoman Empire* (Cambridge: Cambridge University Press, 1997).

—, 'Clothing Laws, State and Society in the Ottoman Empire, 1720–1829', *International Journal of Middle East Studies* (1997), pp. 403–25.

—, *The Ottoman Empire: 1700–1922* (New York: Cambridge University Press, 2000).

Rıza T., *Tıp Fakültesi Tarihçesi: Mir'at-ı Mektebi Tıbbiye* (The History of Faculty of Mecine), ed. A. Kazancıgil (Istanbul: Özel Yayınlar, 1991).

Rublack, U., 'Pregnancy, Childbirth and the Female Body in Early Modern Germany', *Past and Present*, 150 (1996), pp. 84–110.

—, 'The Public Body: Policing Abortion in Early Modern Germany', in L. Abrams and E. Harvey (eds), *Gender Relations in German History: Power, Agency, and Experience from the Sixteenth to the Twentieth Century* (Durham, NC: Duke University Press, 1997), pp. 57–80.

Sakacı, F., *Her Doğum Bir Mucizedir, Aykut Kazancıgil Kitabı* (Every Child Birth is a Miracle, The Book of Aykut Kazancıgil) (Istanbul: İş Kültür Yayınları, 2005).

Salzmann, A., 'Measures of Empire: Tax Farming and the Ottoman Ancien Regime, 1695–1807' (PhD dissertation, Columbia University, 1995).

—, 'Citizens in Search of a State: The Limits of Political Participation in the Late Ottoman Empire' in M. Hanagan and C. Tilly (eds), *Extending Citizenship, Reconfiguring States* (New York: Rowman and Littlefield Publishers, 1999), pp. 37–66.

Sarı, N., 'Osmanlı Sağlık Hayatında Kadının Yeri' (The Place of Women in Ottoman Health), *New History of Medicine Studies*, 2–3 (1996–7), pp. 11–64.

—, 'Osmanlı Sağlık Hayatında Kadının Yerine Kısa bir Bakış' (A Brief Overview of the Place of Women in Ottoman Health) in N. Yıldırım (ed.), *Sağlık Alanında Türk Kadını :Cumhuriyetin ve Tıp Fakültesine Kız Öğrenci Kabulünün 75. Yılı* (Turkish Women in the Field of Health: The 75th Anniversary of the Republics and the Admission of Female Students to the Faculty of Medicine) (Istanbul: Novartis, 1998), pp. 166–86.

Sarıyıldız, G., *Hicaz Karantina Teşkilatı: 1865–1914* (Hejaz Quarantine Organization) (Ankara: Türk Tarih Kurumu, 1996).

Saygılıgil, F., 'Osmanlı'da Sağlık Alanında Tedavi Gören ve Tedavi Eden Olarak Kadınlar' (Women as Providers and Receivers of Health Services in the Ottoman Health Sector) , in A. İlyasoğlu and N. Akgökçe (eds), *Yerli Bir Feminizme Doğru* (Towards a Local Feminism) (Istanbul: Sel, 2001), pp. 127–54.

Schick, I. C., 'Print Capitalism and Women's Sexual Agency in the Late Ottoman Empire', *Comparative Studies of South Asia, Africa and the Middle East*, 31:1 (2011), pp. 196–216.

Schiebinger, L., *Nature's Body: Gender in the Making of Modern Science* (Boston, MA: Beacon Press, 1993).

Schlumbohm, J., '"The Pregnant Women are here for the Sake of the Teaching Institution": The Lying-in Hospital of Gottingen University, 1751 to *c.* 1830', *Social History of Medicine*, 14:1 (2001), pp. 59–78.

Scott, J. C., *Seeing Like a State: How Certain Schemes to Improve the Human Condition Have Failed* (New Haven, CT: Yale University Press, 1998).

Sehsuvaroğlu, B., 'Doğumun Tarihçesine ve Bizde Ebelik Öğretimine bir Bakış' (An Approach to Our History of Childbirth and the Midwifery Education), *Türk Jinekoloji ve Obstetrik Mecmuası* (Turkish Journal of Gynaecology and Obstetrics), 4 (1967), pp. 3–4.

Semerdjian, E., *"Off the Straight Path": Illicit Sex, Law, and Community in Ottoman Aleppo* (Syracuse, NY: Syracuse University Press, 2008).

Sener, A., *Tanzimat Dönemi Osmanlı Vergi Sistemi* (Ottoman System of Taxation during Tanzimat Period) (Istanbul: İşaret Yayınları, 1990).

Sezenel, K. T., 'Prof. General Besim Ömer Akalın'ın Ölümü' (The Death of Prof. General Besim Ömer Akalın), *Türk Ginekoloji Arşivi*, 4–25 (1940), pp. 1174–6.

Shaw, S. J., 'The Nineteenth-Century Ottoman Tax Reforms and Revenue System', *International Journal of Middle East Studies*, 6:4 (1975), pp. 421–59.

Simsek, E., 'Çukurova'da Anlatılan 'Alkarısı' Efsanelerinin Türk Efsaneleri İçindeki Yeri' (The Place of 'Alkarısı' Legent [and Mythologies of Childbirth] among the Turkish Mythologies), in *I. Uluslararası Karacaoğlan ve Çukurova Halk Kültürü Sempozyumu (21–23 Kasım 1990, Adana)–Bildiriler* (The First International Symposium on Karacaoglan and Cukurova Local Culture) (Adana, 1991).

Simşek, F, H. Eroğlu and G. Dinç, 'Osmanlı İmparatorluğunda Iskat-ı Cenin (Çocuk Düşürme)' (Abortion in the Ottoman Empire), in *Uluslararası Sosyal Araştırmalar Dergisi/Journal of International Social Research*, 2:6 (2009), pp. 593–609.

Somel, S. A., 'Osmanlı Reform Çağında Osmanlıcılık Düşüncesi (1839–1913)' (The Idea of Ottomanism in the Age of Ottoman Reform (1839-1913)), in M. Belge (ed.), *Modern Türkiye'de Siyasi Düşünce: Tanzimat ve Cumhuriyet'in Birikimi* (The Political Ideas in Modern Turkey: The Accumulations of Tanzimat and the Republic) (Istanbul: İletişim Yayınevi, 2001).

—, *The Modernization of Public Education in the Ottoman Empire: 1839–1908 Islamization, Autocracy and Discipline* (Leiden: Brill, 2001).

—, 'Osmanlı Son Döneminde Iskat-ı Cenin Meselesi' (Abortion in the Late Ottoman Period), *Kebikeç*, 13 (2002), pp. 65–88.

—, 'The Issue of Abortion in 19th Century Ottoman Empire', in H. İnalcık and O. Özel (eds), *IXth International Congress of Economic and Social History of Turkey Dubrovnik-Croatia, 20–23, 2002* (Ankara: Atatürk Supreme Council for Culture, Language & History, Publications of the Turkish Historical Society, 2005), pp. 339–46.

—, 'Sources on the Education of Ottoman Women in the Prime Ministerial Ottoman Archive for the Period of Reforms in the Nineteenth and Early Twentieth Centuries', in A. A. Sonbol (ed.), *Beyond the Exotic: Women's Histories in Islamic Societies* (Syracuse, NY: Syracuse University Press, 2005), pp. 295–306.

Sonbol, A. A. (ed.), *Women, the Family, and Divorce Laws in Islamic History* (Syracuse, NY: Syracuse University Press, 1996).

Süheyl, A., *Besim Ömer Paşa ve Doğum Tarihi* (Besim Ömer Paşa and the History of Childbirth) (Istanbul: Ahmet İhsan Matbaası, 1932).

Sunar, M., 'Cauldron of Dissent: A Study of the Janissary Corps, 1807–1826' (PhD dissertation, Binghamton University, 2007).

Szreter, S., *Fertility, Class and Gender in Britain, 1860–1940* (Cambridge: Cambridge University Press, 1996).

Taner, T., 'Tanzimat Devrinde Ceza Hukuku' (The Criminal Law during the Tanzimat Period) , in *Tanzimat* (Istanbul, 1940), pp. 226–30.

Taşkıran, N., *Haseki'nin Kitabı: İstanbul Haseki Külliyesi* (The Book of Haseki: Istanbul Haseki Complex) (Istanbul: Haseki Hastanesini Kalkındırma Derneği, 1972).

—, 'Türkiye'de Ebelik Eğitimi' (The Midwifery Education in Turkey), *Haseki Tıp Bülteni* (Haseki Bulletin of Medicine), 2:3 (1973), pp. 229–40.

Tatlock, L., 'Speculum Feminarum: Gendered Perspectives on Obstetrics and Gynecology in Early Modern Germany', *Signs*, 17:4 (1992), pp. 725–60.

Tuchman, A. M., '"The True Assistant to the Obstetrician": State Regulation and the Legal Protection of Midwives in Nineteenth Century Prussia', *Social History of Medicine*, 18:1 (2005), pp. 23–38.

Tucker, J. E., and M. Meriwether (eds), *Social History of Women and Gender in the Modern Middle East* (Boulder, CO: Westview Press, 1999).

Tuğ, B., 'Politics of Honor: The Institutional and Social Frontiers of "Illicit" Sex in Mid-Eighteenth-Century Ottoman Anatolia' (PhD dissertation, New York University, 2009).

Turna, N., 'Pandemonium and Order: Suretyship, Surveillance, and Taxation in Early Nineteenth-Century Istanbul', *New Perspectives on Turkey*, 39 (Fall 2008), pp. 167–89.

Ulman, Y. I., 'Journal de Constantinople'a göre Mekteb-i Tıbbiye-i Adliye-i Şahane'nin Galatasaray Dönemi' (The Galatasaray Period of The Imperial School of Medicine According to the Journal de Constantinople) (MA Thesis, Istanbul University, 1994).

—, 'Mecmua-i Fünun'da Tıp Konulu Yazılar' (The Articles on Medicine in Mecmua-i Fünun), *Bilim Tarihi* (History of Science), 22 (1993), pp. 17–30.

—, 'Besim Ömer Akalın (1820–1940): Ange Gardien des Femmes et des Enfants', in M. Anastasiadou-Dumont (ed.), *Medecins et ingenieurs Ottomans à l'age des nationalismes* (Paris: Maisonneuve et Larose; Institut Français d'Etudes Anatoliennes, 2003).

—, 'Osmanlıdan Cumhuriyete Geçiş Sürecinde Bir Aydın Portresi: Besim Ömer Akalın' (A Portrait of an Intellectual during the Process of Transition from the Ottoman Period to the Republic), *Müteferrika*, 25 (2004).

Ulrich, L. T., '"The Living Mother of a Living Child": Midwifery and Mortality in Post-Revolutionary New England', *William and Mary Quarterly*, 46:1 (1989), pp. 27–48.

—, *A Midwife's Tale: The Life of Martha Ballard, Based on her Diary, 1785–1812* (New York: Knopf, 1990).

Uludağ, O. Ş., *Beşbuçuk Asırlık Türk Tababeti Tarihi* (The History of Five Hundred and Fifty Years of Turkish Medicine) (Ankara: Kültür Bakanlığı, 1991).

Unat, E. K., and M. Samasti, *Mekteb-i Tıbbiye-i Mülkiye (Sivil Tıp Mektebi) 1867–1909* (The Civil School of Medicine) (Istanbul, 1990).

Unver, A. S., *Haseki Hastanesi Tarihçesi: 400. Yıldönümü Dolayısıyla* (The History of Haseki Hospital: In Its 400th Anniversary) (Istanbul: İstanbul Üniversitesi Tıp Tarihi Enstitüsü, 1939).

—, Tarihte Ebeler ve Doğum Tarihimiz' (Midwives in History and Our History of Childbirth), *II. Ana Sağlığı Semineri* (The Second Seminar on Mothers' Health) (Istanbul, 1967).

Usborne, C, 'Abortion for Sale! The Competition Between Quacks and Doctors in Weimar Germany', in M. Gijswit-Hofstra, H. Marland and H. Vaard (eds), *Illness and Healing Alternatives in Western Europe* (London: Routledge, 1997), pp. 183–204.

—, 'Wise Women, Wise Men and Abortion in the Weimar Republic: Gender, Class and Medicine', in L. Abrams and E. Harvey (eds), *Gender Relations in German History: Power, Agency, and Experience from the Sixteenth to the Twentieth Century* (Durham, NC: Duke University Press, 1997).

Ustünel, B. and E. Bayırlı, 'Ebelik ve Tarihi Gelişimi' (Midwifery and Its Progress), *Zeynep Kamil Tıp Bülteni* (Zeynep Kamil Bulletin of Medicine), 3:2 (1971), pp. 67–74.

—, 'Ebelik ve Tarihi Gelişimi'(Midwifery and Its Progress), *Zeynep Kamil Tıp Bülteni* (Zeynep Kamil Bulletin of Medicine), 3:3 (1971), pp. 209–16.

—, 'Ebelik ve Tarihi Gelişimi'(Midwifery and Its Progress), *Zeynep Kamil Tıp Bülteni* (Zeynep Kamil Bulletin of Medicine), 4:1 (1972), pp. 1–6.

Voss, L. H. V., 'Introduction', *International Review of Social History*, 46 (2001), pp. 1–10.

Wiesner, M., 'The Midwives of South Germany and the Public/Private Dichotomy', in H. Marland (ed.), *The Art of Midwifery: Early Modern Midwives in Europe* (London: Routledge, 1994), pp. 77–94.

Wishnitzer, A., 'The Transformation of Ottoman Temporal Culture During the "Long Nineteenth Century"' (Unpublished PhD dissertation, Tel Aviv University, 2009).

Yıldırım, N. (ed.), 'Tanzimat'tan Cumhuriyet'e Koruyucu Sağlık Uygulamaları' (The Protective practices of Health from Tanzimat to the Republic), in *Tanzimat'tan Cumhuriyet'e Türkiye Ansiklopedisi* (Encyclopaedia of Turkey from Tanzimat to the Republic), 6 vols (Istanbul: İletişim Yayınevi, 1985), vol. 5, pp. 1320–38.

—, *Sağlık Alanında Türk Kadını: Cumhuriyetin ve Tıp Fakültesine Kız Öğrenci Kabulünün 75. Yılı* (Turkish Women in the Field of Health: The 75th Anniversary of the Republics and the Admission of Female Students to the Faculty of Medicine) ((Istanbul: Novartis, 1998), pp. 166–86.

—, 'Kadınların Hekim Olma Mücadelesi' (The Struggle of Women to be Doctors), *Toplumsal Tarih* (Social History), 147 (2006), pp. 50–7.

—, 'Osmanlı Coğrafyasında Karantina Uygulamalarına İsyanlar, Karantina İstemezuk' (The Opposition to the Practices of Quarantine in Ottoman Geography, We Do Not Want Quarantine), *Toplumsal Tarih* (Social History), 150 (2006), pp. 18–27.

—, 'Sabuncuoğlu Şerafeddin', *Türkiye Diyanet Vakfı İslam Ansiklopedisi* , 41 vols (Turkish Foundation of Religion Encyclopaedia of Islam), 35 (Istanbul: Türkiye Diyanet Vakfı, 2008), pp. 358–9.

Yılmaz, C., and N. Yılmaz (eds), *Osmanlılarda Sağlık* (Health in the Ottomans) (Istanbul: Biofarma İlaç Sanayi ve Ticaret A.Ş., 2006).

Yosmaoğlu, İ. K., 'Counting Bodies, Shaping Souls: The 1903 Census and National Identity in Ottoman Macedonia', *International Journal of Middle East Studies*, 38 (2006), pp. 55–77.

Zarinebaf-Shahr, F., 'Women, Patronage and Charity in Ottoman İstanbul', in A. A. Sonbol (ed.), *Beyond the Exotic: Women's Histories in Islamic Societies* (Syracuse, NY: Syracuse University Press, 2005).

—, *Crime and Punishment in Istanbul, 1700–1800* (Berekely, CA: University of California Press, 2010).

Ze'evi, D., 'Women in 17th-Century Jerusalem: Western and Indigenous Perspectives', *International Journal of Middle East Studies*, 27:2 (1995), pp. 157–73.

—, 'The Use of Ottoman Sharia Court Records as a Source for Middle Eastern Social History: A Reappraisal', *Islamic Law and Society*, 5:1 (1998), pp. 35–56.

—, *Producing Desire: Changing Sexual Discourse in the Ottoman Middle East, 1500–1900* (Berkeley, CA: University of California Press, 2006).

Zilfi, M. (ed.), *Women in the Ottoman Empire: Middle Eastern Women in the Early Modern Era* (Leiden: Brill, 1997).

Zürcher, E. J., *Arming the State: Military Conscription in the Middle East and Central Asia, 1775–1925* (London: I. B. Tauris, 1999).

INDEX

For Product Safety Concerns and Information please contact our EU
representative GPSR@taylorandfrancis.com
Taylor & Francis Verlag GmbH, Kaufingerstraße 24, 80331 München, Germany

www.ingramcontent.com/pod-product-compliance
Ingram Content Group UK Ltd.
Pitfield, Milton Keynes, MK11 3LW, UK
UKHW011015180926
475701UK00004B/751

* 9 7 8 1 1 3 8 6 6 2 0 0 1 *